Care of the Adult with Intellectual Disability in Primary Care

AN ADAPTATION OF *MANAGEMENT GUIDELINES: DEVELOPMENTAL DISABILITY, VERSION 2* (2005) THERAPEUTIC GUIDELINES LTD

Edited by

PETER LINDSAY

General Practitioner
Thakur Practice, Leeds
RCGP Curriculum Guardian for Intellectual Disability

Foreword by

JILL MORRISON

Professor of General Practice
Dean for Learning and Teaching
College of Medicine, Veterinary Medicine and Life
University of Glasgow

Radcliffe Publishing
London • New York

Radcliffe Publishing Ltd
33–41 Dallington Street
London
EC1V 0BB
United Kingdom

www.radcliffepublishing.com
Electronic catalogue and worldwide online ordering facility.

British Library Cataloguing in Publication Data

A catalogue record for this book is available from the British Library.

ISBN-13: 978 184619 479 5

The paper used for the text pages of this book is FSC® certified. FSC (The Forest Stewardship Council®) is an international network to promote responsible management of the world's forests.

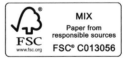

MIX
Paper from
responsible sources
FSC® C013056

Typeset by Pindar NZ, Auckland, New Zealand
Printed and bound by TJI Digital, Padstow, Cornwall, UK

Contents

Foreword

People with intellectual disabilities account for over 2% of our population and for a substantial amount of our work in general practice. Due to improvements in survival at all ages, the proportion of our population living with intellectual disabilities is increasing. The closure over the last few decades of the large institutions, which previously cared for people with intellectual disabilities, means that more patients with intellectual disabilities are now living in the community in a range of circumstances, including supported living arrangements with paid or family carers, or independently.

People with intellectual disabilities are doubly disadvantaged: firstly, by their disabilities; and, secondly, by a healthcare system that is not as flexible or well adapted to meet their needs as it should be. People with intellectual disabilities have the same right to comprehensive healthcare as anyone else. Their right to care includes, for example, preventive healthcare and yet rates of screening in this group are much lower than for the general population.

As GPs, we have a duty to ensure that everybody has equitable access to primary healthcare. This may mean that special arrangements are required to ensure that people who can't tell the time can attend booked appointments in our surgeries, or that people who are too restless to wait have the first appointment, or extra time is allocated to people who have communication difficulties. Practices that are organised in a way that enables equity of access for people with intellectual disabilities are likely to be providing very high standards of care for all of their patients.

The role of the GP in looking after people with intellectual disabilities is basically the same as our role in managing the general population and includes screening, diagnosing and treating new health problems, managing long-term conditions, referring where appropriate and so on. People with intellectual disabilities experience the range of problems found in the general population but sometimes in a differing pattern of risk. For example, epilepsy, visual and hearing problems, gastro-oesophageal reflux disease, osteoporosis, mental health problems and abuse are all more common. As the first point of contact for people with intellectual disabilities with health services, we in primary care need to be aware of the presentations and particular needs of this group. This book is a very welcome review of the physical, psychological and social problems and issues experienced by people with intellectual disabilities, which we need to be familiar with to provide high quality care and begin to reverse the inequalities in healthcare experienced by this group.

Professor Jill Morrison
Professor of General Practice
Dean for Learning and Teaching
College of Medicine, Veterinary Medicine and Life
University of Glasgow
January 2011

Preface

The publication of the first edition of *Management Guidelines: People with Developmental and Intellectual Disabilities* marked a small but significant step in increasing the recognition of these disabilities within the health professions in Australia and worldwide. It offered in a single volume, for the first time, an approach to healthcare that incorporates the biological, psychological and social aspects of care of adults with intellectual disability. Although people with intellectual disability represent 2% of the population of the developed world – the majority of whom experience poor health and inadequate healthcare – they have received scant attention in the health literature or mainstream press. General practitioners (GPs), who are central to the care of people with intellectual disability, now have to respond to those health needs and this requires combined input from a range of medical and non-medical professions, and most importantly requires the involvement of those with the disability and their carers. The publication of the first edition sought to empower people with intellectual disability, their families and carers, as well as health professionals, to seek and deliver better health and healthcare.

The Royal College of General Practitioners (RCGP) special interest group was therefore delighted when, in the year the Department of Health formally recognised the value of annual health checks for adults with intellectual disability, Radcliffe arranged for the second edition to be published in the UK with sections adapted to the specific need of UK practitioners. Sections referring to legal aspects, autism spectrum conditions and social care have been rewritten and Graham Martin can rejoice that his chapter on annual health checks marks the success of his, at one time, one-man campaign. Many healthcare issues for people with intellectual disability can be dealt with in the same manner as in those without disability so we highlight areas where management differs from that of the general population as the result of the different and idiosyncratic morbidity and mortality suffered by this special population. Aspects that may require a more focused approach are also described.

Matt Hoghton has provided us with the RCGP e-learning section and our nursing colleagues have developed a practical text with their *Oxford Handbook* and this volume and those complement each other and offer GP registrars and all established general practitioners a sound practical basis to practise in this new speciality which 'Valuing People', the Quality Outcomes Framework, 'Health for All' and annual health checks have confirmed is our responsibility.

The resulting text forms a basis for management of patients, but there may be sound clinical reasons for different therapy. The complexity of clinical practice requires that, in all cases, users understand the individual clinical situation, and exercise independent professional judgement. The text has been prepared and revised by an expert group of experienced clinicians and further revised to adapt it to current practice in the UK. It represents an independent consensus distillation and interpretation of the best available evidence and opinion at the time of publication and is the first benchbook referring to the medical care of adults with intellectual disability in the UK. Its development from an Australian text has enabled us to make it available early in the development of annual health checks but it will, without doubt, need revising and improving.

The original editorial board and the RCGP special interest group hope this book allows those of you with intellectual disability to gain better health, or if you are caring for a person affected, that it creates more positive health results. For the clinicians using this book, we trust it will support your practice and help and encourage you to develop annual health checks and other services in your day-to-day practice and improve the health outcomes for this previously overlooked minority to whom we provide care.

For the sake of the ISBN there is a single Editor, but this volume is the result of a team effort of all the RCGP special interest group with support and involvement being given unstintingly for all. Dr Ian White deserves his special mention in the front pages and I, as always, acknowledge the support of the Thakur Practice and of my two daughters whose love and comfort kept me going through the dark days of my career and made the brighter days even brighter.

For the next edition we all hope to see, we welcome any further endorsements and any criticisms, comments or rewritten chapters – please contact us via Radcliffe Publishing.

Peter Lindsay
January 2011

COMPLEMENTARY RESOURCES

- Gates B, Barr O. *Oxford Handbook of Learning and Intellectual Disability Nursing*. Oxford: OUP; 2009.
- RCGP. *e-Learning for General Practice. Care of the adult with learning disability*. London: RCGP; 2009. Available at: www.rcgp.org.uk/learningdisabilities (accessed 2 February 2011).

RCGP Intellectual Disability Special Interest Group – core membership

*We remember, first, Dr Ian White who was a resolute member of the
group up to his death in 2009. He was a kind doctor, a good man and a
wonderful father.*
RIP

- **Dr Umesh Chauhan**, Clinical Research Fellow, University of Manchester
- **Dr Matt Hoghton**, RCGP CIRC Clinical Champion for Intellectual Disability
- **Dr Tom Howseman**, GP Champion for Learning Disabilities,
  Northamptonshire
- **Professor Amanda Kirby**, Director of The Dyscovery Centre, University of
  Wales, Newport
- **Dr Peter Lindsay**, GP (Thakur Practice, Leeds), RCGP Curriculum Guardian
  for Intellectual Disability
- **Dr Graham Martin**, GP and first Chairman of Group
- **Dr Jill Rasmussen**, GPwSi Surrey PCT, Chair

Legal Adviser: Kate Banerjee, Solicitor at Jones Myers LLP, Family Law specialists.
In the preparation for the chapter on legal issues she was helped and advised by
Andrew Fox, Barrister at Law, Jones Myers LLP.

TERMS OF REFERENCE OF GROUP
- To develop good practice frameworks for the management of adults with
  intellectual disability including equity of access and the means of developing
  good quality care in the context of the primary healthcare team.
- To develop educational materials for practitioners and those training for
  general practice.
- To set evidence-based quality standards for the care of adults with intellectual
  disability which they and their carers could expect.

Acknowledgements

STEERING GROUP: *MANAGEMENT GUIDELINES: DEVELOPMENTAL DISABILITY, VERSION 2* (2005) THERAPEUTIC GUIDELINES LTD

- **Associate Professor N Lennox** (Chairman and Medical Editor), Director, Queensland Centre for Intellectual and Developmental Disability, University of Queensland
- **Dr H Beange**, Clinical Lecturer, Centre for Developmental Disability Studies, Royal Rehabilitation Centre, Sydney
- **Associate Professor R Davis**, Director, Centre for Developmental Disability Health Victoria, Monash University, Victoria
- **Dr S Durvasula**, Lecturer in Developmental Disability, Centre for Developmental Disability Studies, Faculty of Medicine, University of Sydney
- **Ms N Edwards**, Lecturer and Clinical Coordinator, Queensland Centre for Intellectual and Developmental Disability, University of Queensland
- **Dr P Graves**, Head, Developmental Disabilities Clinic, Monash Medical Centre; Senior Lecturer, Department of Paediatrics, Monash University, Victoria
- **Dr J Maxwell**, Senior Medical Officer, Intellectual Disability Services Council, South Australia
- **Ms J McDowell**, Editor, Therapeutic Guidelines Ltd, Victoria
- **Dr C Mohr**, Consultant Clinical Psychologist, Mental Health Intellectual Disability Team, New Zealand
- **Dr J Torr**, Senior Lecturer and Consultant Psychiatrist, Centre for Developmental Disability Health Victoria, Monash University, Victoria
- **Dr P White**, Research Psychiatrist, Policy and Economics Group, Queensland Centre for Mental Health Research, The Park Centre for Mental Health Treatment, Research and Education

MAJOR CONTRIBUTORS: *MANAGEMENT GUIDELINES: DEVELOPMENTAL DISABILITY, VERSION 2* (2005) THERAPEUTIC GUIDELINES LTD

The Steering Group gives special acknowledgement to the following authors for their major contributions to *Management Guidelines: Developmental Disability*.

- **Professor C Bower**, Senior Principal Research Fellow, Centre for Child

Health Research, University of Western Australia; Institute for Child Health Research, Western Australia

➤ **Dr M Burbidge**, Senior Lecturer, Centre for Developmental Disability Health Victoria, Monash University, Victoria

➤ **Ms J Butler**, Health Educator and Human Relations Consultant, Centre for Developmental Disability Health Victoria, Monash University, Victoria

➤ **Dr A Churchyard**, Consultant Neurologist, Monash Medical Centre, Victoria

➤ **Mr J Cockerill**, Solicitor, Adult Guardian for Queensland (retired), Queensland

➤ **Dr J Cohen**, Senior Lecturer, Department of General Practice, Monash University; Medical Director, Fragile X Alliance Clinic, Victoria

➤ **Dr N Cooling**, Senior Medical Educator, General Practice Training Tasmania, Tasmania

➤ **Dr M Cuskelly**, Co-Director, Down Syndrome Research Program, School of Education, University of Queensland

➤ **Ms J Diggens**, Clinical Psychologist, ParaQuad Victoria; Research Assistant, Department of General Practice, University of Melbourne, Victoria

➤ **Dr G Eastgate**, Senior Lecturer, Queensland Centre for Intellectual and Developmental Disability, University of Queensland

➤ **Dr D Harley**, Senior Lecturer, Queensland Centre for Intellectual and Developmental Disability, University of Queensland

➤ **Ms B Hemsley**, Clinical Educator and Speech Pathologist, University of Sydney, New South Wales

➤ **Dr D Henderson**, GP Educator, Centre for Developmental Disability Health Victoria, Monash University, Victoria

➤ **Dr T Iacono**, Senior Research Fellow, Centre for Developmental Disability Health Victoria, Monash University, Victoria

➤ **Associate Professor N Kerse**, Director of Research, Department of General Practice and Primary Health Care, School of Population Health, University of Auckland, New Zealand

➤ **Dr P King**, Special Needs Dentist, Staff Specialist, Hunter Oral Health Service and Westmead Centre for Oral Health, New South Wales

➤ **Mr F Lambrick**, Senior Clinician, Statewide Forensic Service, Department of Human Services, Victoria

➤ **Dr H Leonard**, Senior Research Fellow, Telethon Institute for Child Health, Western Australia

➤ **Dr J Marshall**, Senior Medical Adviser, Child and Community Health Directorate, Department of Health, Western Australia

➤ **Dr A McElduff**, Senior Staff Specialist, Department of Endocrinology, Royal North Shore Hospital, New South Wales

➤ **Dr A Nielsen**, Consultant Psychiatrist, Queensland Centre for Intellectual and Developmental Disability, University of Queensland

➤ **Dr M Nugent**, Medical Officer, IDSC Strathmont Centre, Adelaide; General Practitioner, Clare Medical Centre, South Australia

➤ **Ms C O'Leary**, Senior Policy Officer, Child and Community Health, Department of Health, Government of Western Australia, Western Australia

➤ **Dr D Palmer**, Medical Director, Choices Clinic, Royal Women's Hospital; Consultant Gynaecologist, Kew Residential Centre, Victoria

- ➤ **Professor D Ravine**, Chair in Medical Genetics, Western Australian Institute for Medical Research, School of Medicine and Pharmacology, University of Western Australia
- ➤ **Associate Professor D Reddihough**, Department of Child Development and Rehabilitation, Royal Children's Hospital, Murdoch Children's Research Institute and University of Melbourne, Victoria
- ➤ **Dr M Rowell**, Consultant Paediatrician, Department of Child Development and Rehabilitation, Royal Children's Hospital, Victoria
- ➤ **Ms L Stewart**, Dietitian-Nutritionist, Bankstown Health Service, New South Wales
- ➤ **Ms M Taylor**, formerly of the Queensland Centre for Intellectual and Developmental Disability, University of Queensland
- ➤ **Professor B Tonge**, Head, School of Psychology, Psychiatry & Psychological Medicine, Monash University; Head, Centre for Developmental Psychiatry & Psychology, Monash University, Monash Medical Centre, Victoria
- ➤ **Dr J Tracy**, Educational Director, Centre for Developmental Disability Health Victoria, Monash University, Victoria
- ➤ **Dr M Tucker**, Lecturer, Queensland Centre for Intellectual and Developmental Disability, University of Queensland

Part One

Overview of intellectual disability care

CHAPTER 1

Definitions, epidemiology and health issues

DEFINITIONS

This book and current literature uses the term intellectual disability to refer to those patients who meet the criteria of learning disability as defined by the ISD and DSM:

ICD-10

A condition of arrested or incomplete development of the mind which is especially characterised by impairment of skills manifested during the developmental period contributing to the overall level of intelligence: cognitive, language, motor and social abilities.

DSM-4

- IQ<70
- Onset before age 18 years
- Dysfunction or impairment of:
  — communication
  — self-care
  — home living
  — social and interpersonal skills
  — use of community resources
  — self-direction
  — academic skills
  — work and leisure
  — health and safety.

However, the Department of Health definition of 1998 which referred to 'learning disability' is the most useful:

A significantly reduced ability to understand new or complex information, to learn new skills, with reduced ability to cope independently, starting before adulthood (age 18 years) with a lasting effect on development.
Impaired intelligence.
Impaired social functioning.
Impaired communication.

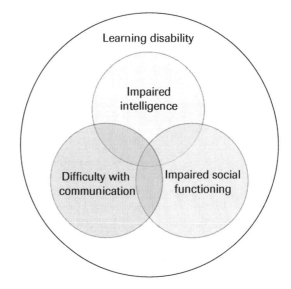

FIGURE 1.1 The triad of intellectual disability

Figure 1.1 illustrates a classical triad everyone can remember in whatever field of medicine they work and might encounter patients with intellectual disability.

Those patients with intellectual disability can be divided into groups according to their IQ, described by ICD-10 and the World Health Organization in 1992:
➤ **Mild** – IQ 50–55 up to 70. This results in independence in social care with ability to maintain social relationships and employment and to learn basic reading and writing skills.
➤ **Moderate** – IQ 35–40 up to 50–55. Adults with this level of disability require additional support in the more complex aspects of modern day life.
➤ **Severe** – IQ 20–25 up to 35–40; **Profound** – IQ<20–25. Adults with this level of disability require a much greater degree of support and have limited communication skills.

Those patients with IQ between 70 and 84 form a little recognised group of 'borderline intelligence' with the following characteristics:
➤ high risk of academic problems
➤ high risk of behavioural problems
➤ visuospatial problems
➤ verbal problems
➤ communication problems
➤ young people with the disorder constitute 80%–90% of their age group serving custodial sentences.

The high risk of being detained in prison suggests it would be cost effective to detect this group early in life and provide active care and support in the same way we are moving to support the slightly more intellectually disabled.

The term 'developmental disability' relates to differences in neurologically based functions that have their onset before birth or during childhood and are associated with significant long-term difficulties. Patients with developmental disability may not have intellectual disability, e.g. those with autism spectrum disorder or some types of cerebral palsy.

Other terms referring to these patients have fallen into disuse, including those derogatory Victorian terms of 'imbecile', 'idiot' and 'feeble minded'. 'Mental deficiency' was used in 1913, 'mental subnormality' in 1959, and 'mental handicap' was commonly used in the 1950s and 1960s by the relatives of patients who did not like the term 'subnormality'. 'Learning disability' was a term used first by the Secretary of State for Health in 1991, but the term 'intellectual disability' is now recognised and used internationally and will be used throughout this book.

For completeness and clarification it is worth listing those patients who do not suffer from intellectual disability:

➤ People who develop an intellectual disability after the age of 18.
➤ People who suffer brain injury in accidents after the age of 18.
➤ People with complex medical conditions which affect their intellectual abilities and which develop after the age of 18, e.g. Huntington's chorea, Alzheimer's disease.
➤ People with specific learning difficulties, e.g. dyslexia, delayed speech and language development, and those with literacy problems – many of whom would fit into the definition of 'Developmental Disability'.

THE SOCIAL MODEL OF DISABILITY

The social model of disability describes how any disability, including intellectual disability, affects the life of an individual depending on:

➤ the severity of the disability
➤ the presence of other disabilities
➤ age
➤ personality and mental health
➤ level of social support
➤ circumstances.

This explains how some well-supported and cared for adults are only detected as having intellectual disability when a crisis which removes that support occurs. For example, Paul has moderate intellectual disability and his parents have a small but successful farm in which Paul has always worked since he left school without any GCSEs. His friends are always welcome and he has a good social life with a regular small twice weekly allowance his dad gives him. When his mum becomes disabled by Parkinson's and his dad goes into hospital, Paul is arrested for driving a hay lorry around the high street with its straw burning.

INCIDENCE AND PREVALENCE

Approximately 2% of the population have intellectual disability with 25% of them having severe or profound disability. A GP practice will have, on average, 40 patients per 2000 of list size, but there is significant variation in the proportion in each practice brought about by the socioeconomic distribution of the practice population, the cost of property in the practice area and the presence of communal living homes in the practice area, which is affected by the cost of property. A practice's enthusiasm in caring for and attitude to patients with intellectual disability affects the way carers register them with a list. There is 'downward pressure' on the incidence, resulting from prenatal diagnosis and improved neonatal care, but also upwards pressure, resulting from older parents having children later in their own lives, greater survival in special care baby units (SCBUs) and improved effectiveness of treatments in the neonatal period and afterwards and the increased incidence of adults with intellectual disability in families in ethnic minorities. In the UK this is likely to mean that between 2001 and 2021 there will be:

➤ 11% increase of adults with intellectual disability
➤ 36% increase of those over 60 years with intellectual disability.

THE SOCIOECONOMIC EFFECTS OF INTELLECTUAL DISABILITY

The origins of intellectual disability are discussed in Chapter 6 but, in general, whereas severe and profound disability are likely to be due to sporadic causes which have equal prevalence in all socioeconomic groups, moderate and mild disability are the result of polygenic inheritance and therefore the patient's relatives are more likely to be similarly affected and, as will be seen, will therefore be in the lower socioeconomic groups as being an adult with intellectual disability or having intellectual disability reduces the overall income of the household. Forty-four per cent of families including an adult or child with learning disability live in poverty compared to 33% of other families. Sixty per cent of 16–19 year olds with intellectual disability do not have education, training or employment. Only 17% of adults with intellectual disability were in paid employment in 2003–04; 20% of men and 47% of women had an unpaid job. Paid employment was more common in:

➤ those receiving less supportive care
➤ those who did not have a long-standing illness or disability
➤ men
➤ those who lived in smaller households
➤ those who saw friends with intellectual disability less often and friends who did not have intellectual disability more often
➤ white Caucasians
➤ those who lived in areas of high employment
➤ those who had good general health.

TRANSFER OF CARE FROM LONG-TERM HOSPITALS

Anyone thinking the Victorians heartless must remember that it was up until the 1980s that patients with intellectual disability were kept in long-stay hospitals walled away from the rest of the community, often from childhood to death. The 1990s saw those hospitals rapidly emptied, as Table 1.1. shows.

TABLE 1.1 1990–2003: changes in residences of adults with intellectual disability in the UK

Own home	200% increase
Family home or foster care	20% increase
Supported living	200% increase
Hospitals/NHS	95% decrease
Local authority	30% decrease
Private	150% increase

MEDICAL CARE

Primary care has had the care of patients with intellectual disability devolved to it. Following the transfer of patients from long-stay hospitals into the community, the psychiatrists responsible for their care attempted in some areas to act as the physician offering total care, but workload pressures and the complexity of the medical care needed led to consideration being given of who was to offer this care, with many position statements and policy documents produced – a sample only is listed in the Further Reading.

The Department of Health policy acknowledges that the complexities of that care and the increasing numbers of patients with learning disability now mean that general practitioners should adopt this central role.

The Department of Health's Quality and Outcomes Framework 2006 was the first official document to infer that the care of the learning disabled had devolved to primary care, by requiring practices to create a register of adults with intellectual disability on the practice register. It followed on the Disability Rights Commission statement of 2006 which highlighted the inadequate care offered to adults with intellectual disability.

The charity Mencap's harrowing report *Death by Indifference*, which included descriptions of care of one young adult who was not given analgesia for a fractured femur for three days and another who was not fed for more than three weeks, led to Sir Michael Joseph's report, *Health For All*, which, among many recommendations:
> ➤ obliged the NHS in all its functions to make 'reasonable adjustment' to the needs of patients with intellectual disability
> ➤ obliged medical education to include care of adults with intellectual disability at undergraduate and postgraduate levels – it is now included in the nMRCGP
> ➤ instructed primary care trusts (PCTs) and strategic health authorities (SHAs) to encourage GPs through Direct Educational Services (DES) funding to offer annual health checks (*see* Chapters 10 and 11) to all adults with intellectual disability.

A DIFFERENT PATTERN OF MORBIDITY AND MORTALITY ASSOCIATED WITH INTELLECTUAL DISABILITY

In general the more severe and profound the intellectual disability the greater the chance the patient will also have associated physical disability. Intellectual disability is associated with an increased (two to three times) incidence of health problems and an idiosyncratic morbidity. An adult with intellectual disability is four times more likely to die of a preventable illness, 58 times more likely to die up to the age of 50 years and two to four times more likely to suffer a long-term chronic illness or disability.

The three principal causes of death are (*see* Chapter 8):
➤ respiratory infections
➤ ischaemic heart disease
➤ upper gastrointestinal malignancies.

In spite of this increased morbidity, increased health needs and increased mortality, repeated studies demonstrated unmet needs. A national review in 2003–04 showed 4% of adults had not seen a GP in the last three years. In Gateshead more than a third of adults with Down syndrome (*see* Chapter 24) had not seen a GP in the last 12 months, less than half of them had been immunised to influenza, none had been immunised to hepatitis B, and there was non-formal screening of thyroid disease, known to be associated with Down syndrome. In another study of women with intellectual disability only 24% had ever had any form of breast examination.

Studies of the health of adults with learning disability have shown an increased incidence of the following.
➤ **Dysphagia**: affecting 5%–8% of adults in the community and 33% of those in hospitals (*see* Chapter 18).
➤ **Hearing problems**: affecting 12% – 40 times that of other adults.
➤ **Vision problems**: affecting 7% – 10 times that of other adults.
➤ **Obesity**: affecting 33% – 1.5 times that of other adults, but 7% suffer from severe obesity and among patients with Down syndrome 75% are obese (*see* Chapter 17).
➤ **Nutritional problems**: these are common, related to dysphasia, gastro-oesophageal reflux disease (GORD), and intrinsic disorders predisposing to obesity, e.g. Prader-Willi syndrome (*see* Chapter 28).
➤ **Epilepsy**: up to 20% affected, which is 20 times that of other adults. The epilepsy is commonly difficult to control and often requires polytherapy. It can present with behaviour problems or psychiatric symptoms.
➤ **Asthma**: twice as common as in other adults.
➤ **Type 2 diabetes**: more common and occurs in younger patients.
➤ **Hypothyroidism**: increased incidence, particularly in adults with Down syndrome (*see* Chapter 24).
➤ **Dental problems**: affecting 86% of any population of adults with intellectual disability (*see* Chapter 19).
➤ **Constipation**: varying rates described but acknowledged as a common problem.
➤ **GORD**: increased incidence associated with dysphasia and increased prevalence of *H. pylori* infection in those adults living in communal homes.
➤ **Osteoporosis**: increased incidence and occurring earlier in life, related to immobility, diet, enzyme-inducing anticonvulsants and early menopause or hypogonadism (*see* Chapters 21 and 22).
➤ **Mental health problems**: (*see* Chapter 14) Alzheimer's disease is more common and occurs earlier in life, especially in patients with Down syndrome.
➤ **Behaviour problems**: (*see* Chapter 12) sometimes related to the cause of the intellectual disability.

In general, intellectual disability is associated with premature ageing – earlier onset Type 2 diabetes, menopause, osteoporosis and Alzheimer's disease.

The reasons for this increased morbidity are unexplained but could be related to the following:

➤ genetic and chromosomal abnormalities which are the cause of the intellectual disability and have affected other body systems
➤ associated physical disabilities such as hypotonia and spinal deformities resulting in dysphagia
➤ personal behaviour, particularly inadequate exercise due to reluctance to use communal gyms or swimming pools
➤ immune deficiencies which are commonly detected in association with intellectual disability
➤ an accelerated ageing process
➤ dysphagia, resulting in an increased incidence of respiratory disorders due to inhalation and upper gastrointestinal malignancies due to stasis
➤ novel diseases associated with the genotype.

Preventive care campaigns rarely involve conditions affecting adults with intellectual disability and so literature such as that produced by Easyhealth (www. easyhealth.org) needs to be distributed instead. Adults with intellectual disability are in need of a proactive influenza/pneumococcal immunisation programme and for those at risk – which means anyone mixing with other adults with intellectual disability – hepatitis B immunisation programme at practice and district level. The high rate of deaths from respiratory disorders indicate the need for an influenza/ pneumococcal campaign, and the high risk of encountering someone with challenging behaviour at a time of impaired immunity makes the hepatitis B vaccine essential.

Many studies have shown that adults admitted to hospital with intellectual disability in the UK are discharged earlier than their counterparts without disability. At the time of admission and during admission the adult with intellectual disability should have a known carer or relative present. Discussions between the hospital team and the primary care team are essential and need to be facilitated and encouraged on both sides. Some consultants have developed an expertise in treating adults with intellectual disability and PCT referral management services need to be advised of this at the time of referral.

DIAGNOSIS OF ACUTE ILLNESS

Adults with intellectual disability presenting with acute illnesses pose particular problems and the following checklist should be considered each time, particularly when the cause of the illness is not immediately clear:

➤ **Severe infection**: this can develop quickly and lead rapidly to septicaemia due to immune system deficiency.
➤ **Heart disease**: ischaemic heart disease can present with 'silent infarcts', heart failure or dysrhythmias. Valvular heart disease can progress rapidly due to associated disorders of collagen.
➤ **Malignancy**: atypical presentations of upper gastrointestinal malignancies and malignancies of the gall-bladder and bile ducts are common.
➤ **Asthma** can present acutely when previously less severe symptoms have been

missed, particularly when the patient has been unable to do peak flow rate (PFR) monitoring.

➤ **Side-effects of drugs**: especially psychotropic agents and polypharmacy.
➤ **Foreign bodies** in various bodily orifices producing confusing complex symptoms.
➤ **Depression**: this is common and can cause severe physical symptoms as well as behavioural problems.
➤ **Physical, sexual and emotional abuse** is common, whether in the home or communal home.

DIAGNOSTIC OVERSHADOWING

In assessing a patient's symptoms when he/she presents with acute or long-standing symptoms mistakes can arise if those symptoms are attributed to the intellectual disability rather than other treatable causes. This is particularly important when the patient presents with a change of behaviour. At all times consideration should be given to potential physical, emotional, social and environmental causes and this can require phoning around various agencies to obtain a full history.

MAKING 'REASONABLE ADJUSTMENT' IN PRIMARY CARE

To be able to offer care to adults with intellectual disability a practice is required to adapt to their needs.

➤ Appointments which do not cause anxiety by long waits in the surgery should be offered at the beginning or end of surgery.
➤ The duration of the consultation usually requires lengthening so that a history and views can be obtained from the patient and from the carer/relative.
➤ Everyone in the practice has to accept that telephone consultations will not be as useful, e-mail is almost useless and electronic patient call devices cause anxiety and may not be fit for purpose.
➤ At times it is useful to discuss with the adult with learning disability who he/she is happy for you to talk with about their problems and record this in the notes so if they become acutely unwell you are at less risk of breaching confidentiality.

Nurses, receptionists and secretaries often have first point of contact with the learning disabled and their carers. As part of practice training and development, these staff need to be made aware that adults with intellectual disability:

➤ commonly have vision and hearing problems
➤ commonly have communication problems
➤ commonly have mobility problems and means of access may need to be modified
➤ present with acute illness in unusual ways
➤ benefit in health and overall well-being from annual health checks.

A National Patient Safety Agency (NPSA) review of the care of adults with intellectual disability concluded that the major factors resulting in poor or inadequate care were:

➤ difficulty obtaining relevant information about patients' previous and present health

➤ inappropriate use of physical intervention
➤ vulnerability in acute hospital settings
➤ misdiagnosis or failure to diagnose illness
➤ dysphagia.

The major contribution a GP can make to the overall care of these patients is to attempt to achieve good communication with the patient and all other professionals involved.

COMMUNICATION WITH THE PATIENT AND OTHERS

Patients with intellectual disability have communication difficulties due to:
➤ higher brain function and cognitive difficulties
➤ hearing and understanding problems
➤ language and phonology problems
➤ associated autism spectrum condition (*see* Chapter 26)
➤ speech difficulties
➤ problems with social interaction
➤ sometimes or present social isolation and previous institutionalisation in long-term hospitals
➤ speech, language and phonology problems resulting from:
  − oropharyngeal anatomy
  − oral hygiene
  − salivation
  − motor disorders
  − central nervous systems (CNS) disorders
  − medication – especially dystonia from psychotropic agents
  − mental health – especially depression.

Providers of healthcare also suffer intrinsic problems with communication.
➤ Time restraints: those with intellectual disability need longer consultations for both history taking and explanation of treatment.
➤ Training: because the majority of this minority were kept outside the mainstream health service there has been little academic study of their physical health and that available is not in mainstream journals and publications. (Martin G).
➤ Experience: for the same reason there are few practitioners with long experience of the care of adults with intellectual disability.
➤ Atypical presentations of a different group of illnesses make usual history taking techniques less useful.
➤ Professional empathy with this group of patients and the policy of the local PCT/SHA obviously will affect the care given as this new facet of primary care develops.

When a GP has seen an adult with learning disability there must be communication:
➤ with the patient
➤ with the carer accompanying the patient; you may need to offer to see the carer alone
➤ with the patient's key worker because he/she may be able to give you a fuller and more useful history

➤ with the patient's family – usually the parents but it may be others; you may need to see the family alone
➤ with all other agencies involved in the care of the patient – training centre staff, community learning disability team, district nurses etc. (*see* Box 1.1).

Communication about each consultation is improved if supporting or related information can be provided.
➤ Using literature such as that available from Easyhealth, which is written in terms that the patient can understand and usually has supporting illustrations.
➤ Leaflets, posters and even videos in the waiting area give the message that you are aware of the special problems facing learning disabled patients and can advise about other locally available services.
➤ Using questionnaires such as Pass-AD or dementia screening tools which prompt the carers to look at certain aspects of behaviour as well as providing you with useful information.
➤ The care of the adult with intellectual disability in non-English speaking communities and ethnic minorities poses considerable difficulties and intensive support from the SHA or PCT is often needed.

BOX 1.1 Agencies sharing care of the adult with intellectual disability with the GP

Psychiatry for the learning disabled team
Psychology for the learning disabled team
District nurse
Community Learning Disability Nursing service
Physiotherapist*
Occupation therapist*
Pharmacist
Speech and language therapist*
Social worker*
Dentist*
Dietician*
Optician
Orthoptist (usually in eye clinic – occasionally in community)
Podiatrist*
Wheelchair clinic
Orthotic and appliances clinic*
Incontinence adviser
Macmillan Nursing Service for end of life care
Hospital specialist clinics relevant to individual patient needs
Benefits adviser
Genetic counselling service – may be relevant to siblings and younger family members of patient

* These may be attached to learning disability services or may be generic services depending on local provision.

When taking a history from parents it is worth considering the following.
➤ Parents sometimes exaggerate the abilities and achievement of their children and the parents of adults with intellectual disability are no exception.
➤ The parents may have intellectual disability too.
➤ It is the GP's duty to treat the patient, not the parents, so avoid getting into continuous conspiracies by giving drugs the parents say are necessary but you know are not clinically indicated.

When taking a history from carers it is worth considering the following.
➤ Remember carers have responsibility for the patient and the others they care for – ensure you are not coaxed into managing a patient in a way solely intended to make the lives of the others cared for easier or the work of the carers easier.
➤ If you cannot immediately talk to the key worker, be prepared to phone around until you get the most accurate history.

In taking a history from either parents or carers consider the following.
➤ The parents or carers are in regular contact with the patient and, if experienced, may be better than you at picking up early signs of illness.
➤ Use questionnaires such as the Pass-AD or Alzheimer's screen in Down syndrome to detect and monitor the progress of psychiatric illness.
➤ Remember the possibility of abuse – physical, emotional and sexual.

TREATING THE WHOLE PATIENT WITH DIGNITY AND UNDERSTANDING

As well as adapting to new consulting skills and techniques, being alert to a different range of morbidity and being vigilant to unusual presentations of acute illness, the GP caring for adults with intellectual disability is required to consider the patient, the illness and its investigation and treatment in terms of its social, psychological and ethical impact. A student expressed this, referring to whether a patient should undergo a heart valve replacement with the requirement of subsequent monitoring of anticoagulation:

> If prescription X, which requires as part of its monitoring a blood test every three months, will provide an extra year of life for a middle-aged adult with severe intellectual disability with an estimated life expectancy of another six years, should it be prescribed, considering that each of the 18 blood tests that the patient is subject to will be approached in the same way most of our patients view colonoscopy without anaesthesia?

Simply because an investigation can be done does not mean it should be done or has to be done; a treatment may be available but it may not be appropriate.

Alternatively, the GP's duty of care must ensure that the patient is not deprived of life experiences – holidays, horse riding or rock climbing – simply because others consider it too risky. We all share a dignity of risk when driving cars, riding bikes, swimming or sailing and intellectual disability should not exclude the patient from these risks.

These ethical dilemmas require the GP to discuss and hear the opinions of everyone involved in the care of the patient: family, carers and therapists. They also mean that to accept the challenge to care for this group of patients – to enter into their world, to bring them into our world, to anticipate and sense their anxieties and to remove distress which begins in isolation, uncertainty and the unknown – we must be the best people and the best doctors we are capable of being. We must ensure the patient receives care appropriate to his/her needs but protect him/her from procedures, care and treatments which would not promote well-being and health in its true overall meaning. This is the challenge now facing us – this is the purpose of the rest of this book. If we achieve it, surely many more patients will benefit!

FURTHER READING

- Ali A, Hassiotis A. Illness in people with intellectual disabilities. Is common, underdiagnosed, and poorly managed. *BMJ.* 2008; **336**: 570–1.
- Baxter H, Lowe K, Houston H, *et al.* Previously unidentified morbidity in patients with intellectual disability. *Br J Gen Pract.* 2006; **56**: 93–8.
- Cooper S-A, Melville C, Morrison J. People with intellectual disabilities. Their health needs differ and need to be recognised and met. *BMJ.* 2004: **329**: 414–15.
- Cooper S-A, Smiley E, Morrison J, *et al.* Mental ill-health in adults with intellectual disabilities: prevalence and associated factors. *Br J Psychiatry.* 2007; **190**: 27–35.
- Department of Health (DH). *Valuing People: a new strategy for learning disability for the 21st century.* London: Department of Health; 2001.
- Department of Health (DH). Adults with learning difficulties in England 2003/2004. Available at: www.dhgov.uk/en/Publications andstatistics-4120033
- Department of Health (DH). Quality and Outcomes Framework. 2004. Available at: www. dh.gov.uk/en/Healthcare/Primarycare/Primarycarecontracting/QOF/DH_4125653 (accessed 2 February 2011).
- Disability Rights Commission. Equal treatment: closing the gap. A formal investigation into the physical health inequalities experienced by people with learning disabilities/mental health problems. 2006. Available at: www.equalityhumanrights.com/Documents/DRC/Policy/mainreportword_healthfi1.doc
- Hollins S, Attard MT, Von Fraunhofer N, *et al.* Mortality in people with learning disability: risks, causes, and death certification findings in London. *Dev Med Child Neurol.* 1998; **40**(1): 50–6.
- Kerr M. Improving the general health of people with learning disabilities. *Adv Psych Treat.* 2004; **10**: 200–6.
- Lindsay P, Burgess D. Care of patients with intellectual or learning disability: no more funding so will there be any change? *Br J General Pract.* 2006; **56**(523): 84.
- McGrother CW, Bhaumik S, Thorp CF, *et al.* Epilepsy in adults with intellectual disabilities: prevalence, associations and service implications. *Seizure.* 2006; **15**: 376–86.
- Martin G. Support for people with learning disabilities: the role of primary care. *Prim Care Comm Psych.* 2005; **10**(4): 133–42.
- Martin G, Lindsay PJ. Dying and living with learning disability: will health checks improve the quality of life? *Br J Gen Pract.* 2008; **59**(564): 480–1.
- Matthews T, Weston N, Baxter H, *et al.* A general practice-based prevalence study of epilepsy among adults with intellectual disabilities and of its association with psychiatric disorder, behaviour disturbance and carer stress. *J Intellect Disabil Res.* 2008; **52**(2): 163–73.
- Melville CA, Hamilton S, Hankey CR, *et al.* The prevalence and determinants of obesity in adults with intellectual disabilities. *Obes Rev.* 2007; **8**: 223–30.

- Mencap. Treat me right! 2004. Available at: www.mencap.org.uk/document.asp?id=316 (accessed 2 February 2011).
- Mencap. Death by indifference. 2007. Available at: www.mencap.org.uk/document.asp?id= 284&audGroup=&subjectLevel2=&subjectId=&sorter=1&origin=pageType&pageType=112 &pageno=&searchPhrase
- Michael, Sir J. Healthcare for all: report of the independent inquiry into access to health-care for people with learning disabilities. 2008. Available online at: www.dh.gov.uk/en/ Publicationsandstatistics/Publications/PublicationsPolicyAndGuidance/DH_099255 (accessed 2 February 2011).
- Morgan CL, Scheepers MIA, Kerr MP. Mortality in patients with intellectual disability and epilepsy. *Curr Opin Psychiatry*. 2001; **14**: 471–5.
- National Patient Safety Agency (NPSA). Understanding the patient safety issues for peo-ple with learning disabilities. 2004. Available at: www.salford-pct.nhs.uk/documents/LD/ NPSAUnderstanding.pdf
- Ouelette-Kuntz H. Understanding health disparities and inequities faced by individuals with intellectual disabilities. *J Appl Res Intellect Disabil*. 2005; **18**: 113–21.
- Rimmer JH, Yamaki K. Obesity and intellectual disability. *Ment Retard Dev Disabil Res Rev*. 2006; **12**: 22–7.
- Straetmans JMJAA, van Schrojenstein Lantman-De Valk HMJ, Schellevis FG, *et al*. Health problems of people with intellectual disabilities: the impact for general practice. *Br J Gen Pract*. 2007; **57**: 64–6.
- Sutherland G, Couch MA, Iacono T. Health issues for adults with developmental disability. *Res Dev Disabil*. 2002; **23**: 422–45.
- Tyrer F, Smith LK, McGrother CW. Mortality in adults with moderate to profound intellectual disability: a population-based study. *J Intellect Disabil Res*. 2007; **51**(7): 520–7.
- van Schrojenstein Lantman-De Valk HMJ. Health in people with intellectual disabilities: cur-rent knowledge and gaps in knowledge. *J Appl Res Intellect Disabil* 2005; **18**: 325–33.
- van Schrojenstein Lantman-De Valk HMJ, Metsemakers JFM, Haveman MJ, *et al*. Health problems in people with intellectual disability in general practice: a comparative study. *Fam Pract*. 2000; **17**(5); 405–7.
- Whitaker S, Read S. The prevalence of psychiatric disorders among people with intellectual disabilities: an analysis of the literature. *J Appl Res Intellect Disabil*. 2006; **19**: 330–45.

CHAPTER 2

Care and the carers and families

A patient with intellectual disability moves from the total dependency of infancy to an independent life but is unable to cope with the more complex aspects of communal living and needs support. Initially, that support is offered by parents and family but as both the patient and family grow older, other carers take more and more responsibility.

In the UK figures obtained about adults with intellectual disability in 2003 showed:
➤ 76% live with parents, 30% of whom are older family carers, with 20% being over 65 years and 10% being over 75 years.
➤ 17% live with other members of the family.

Those with severe and profound intellectual disability have parents and other family carers evenly distributed throughout the socioeconomic groups and they will have a wide variation of intellectual disability. Those adults with mild or moderate learning disability are, because of its polygenic origins, more likely to have parents and relatives with similar levels of disability living in socioeconomic deprivation.

Of the minority who do not live with their families:
➤ 6% live alone.
➤ 4% live with a partner.
➤ only 7% have a child and only half of those go on to parent their own child at home.
➤ 16% live in residential homes in which they are fully supported by carers.
➤ 8% live in supported homes in which they are encouraged to take an active role in making meals, keeping the home tidied, etc. and doing their own shopping.
➤ 3% are in hospital.

Of those who do not live with a family member or parent:
➤ 80% continue to have contact with family.
➤ 33% continue to have contact with friends.
➤ 5% have no contact with friends or family.

In a study in Coventry of 360 adults with intellectual disability:
➤ 336 were single.
➤ 18 were married.

➤ 5 were divorced/separated/widowed.
➤ 1 was in a long-term relationship.

These figures suggest that we have a long way to go in offering to adults with intellectual disability a full menu of human activity and interrelationships. We have been set ideals, as with the Declaration of Rights of Disabled Persons by the United Nations in 1975:

> Disabled people, whatever the origin, nature or seriousness of their handicaps and disabilities, have the same fundamental rights as their fellow citizens of the same age, which implies first and foremost the right to enjoy a decent life, as normal and full as possible . . . to be loved and accepted . . . to enjoy companionship . . . to express human emotions . . .

However, this has been difficult as we have tried to unravel the attitudes of society that developed and were unquestioned while so many suffering intellectual disability were segregated from us in long-term hospitals (*see* Chapter 20).

TRANSITIONS FACING PARENTS OF ADULTS WITH INTELLECTUAL DISABILITY

The parents (often elderly) of a patient with intellectual disability have already faced a different series of transitions to other parents:
➤ being told they have an intellectually disabled child
➤ finding a suitable school for the child
➤ negotiating the transition from adolescence to adulthood.

And as their children get older they have to cope with further transitions:
➤ coping with the son or daughter leaving home and often moving to supported living away from the parents
➤ coping with crises in health and bereavement – their own or their adult son/daughter.

FAMILY CARE OF THE ADOLESCENT WITH INTELLECTUAL DISABILITY

The transition from adolescence to adulthood has been described as 'a great abyss' or 'falling off a cliff into a great chasm' and not only is the change dramatic but there is little preparation for it (Department of Health 2001). Up to the age of 16 (or 18 in some areas) the care of the patient is supervised by community paediatricians, with a wide range of specialist services available through that single point of contact. In adulthood it is expected that the intellectually disabled patient will access mainstream health services from an equally wide range of points of contact. Recently, the development of community learning disabled teams has offered a more 'one-stop' support but care is still, in general, fragmented.

SUPPORTING FAMILY CARERS OF THE ADULT WITH INTELLECTUAL DISABILITY

The GP now has the role, which was fulfilled earlier in the patient's life by the community paediatrician, in advocating on behalf of the patient and his/her family to ensure adequate facilities and support. This should include the following.

➤ Respite care, which can take the form of paid carers coming into the home while the parents go out, short breaks with other families or regular stays in communal homes or residential homes that can act as an introduction of the young adult to communal living and the parents to their child gaining 'independence'. One parent described this: 'From when she was 30 she went four times a year for respite care and really liked it and she said she would like to live there. When she was offered a place we could not find a way to let her go as we loved her so much. We were feeling selfish and not letting her go – we realised this in the end and put her name down again and when the next vacancy came up we accepted it'.

➤ Regular occupational therapy and physiotherapy assessments as the adolescent becomes an adult so that walking aids, wheelchairs, bath and toileting aids and hoists are continually adapted to meet the changing circumstances.

➤ Supporting the family in appeals for funding for major structural changes to the home to ensure they can continue to offer safe care.

➤ Advice on benefits. Referral to and liaison with a benefits adviser is essential in this respect, but the GP is often called on to supply medical evidence. This is most common in applications for the Disability Living Allowance as, on first application, many adults without physical disorders but with intellectual disability are refused the mobility component because it is clear they can easily walk more than 50 metres. Medical evidence is required to clarify that while he/she *can* walk the required distance this does not mean he/she *should* do so without the company of a carer or member of the family.

➤ Support when the family carers become unwell. Some suggest that family carers should carry a 'carer's card' describing the problems facing the adults they care for so that if they are taken ill away from home – in shops, benefits offices, etc. – action will be taken to ensure the cared for adult receives continuing care. A GP is in the ideal situation for discussing with the adult with intellectual disability and the older family carers what should happen if one of the carers becomes unwell.

➤ Regular reviews of the health of the parents or other family carers. All reviews stress how physically, mentally and emotionally demanding caring is, resulting in an increased incidence of psychiatric and physical illness among the carers. Carers often put their health needs off, prioritising those of the person they care for. The concept of 'carers' health checks' is coming to primary care whereby carers are offered regular checks of health and reviews of their own long-term health problems at times which fit in with them and those they care for.

➤ Bereavement care when the son or daughter they have been caring for dies. This aspect of bereavement care has received inadequate study and now there are inadequate resources for those affected. I have been with families in which an adult with intellectual disability has died and at no other time have felt so inadequate. Most older family carers spend each day caring for someone they hope will die before them so that they will know he/she has had the best of care. There is therefore a dichotomy of feelings when death does come: 'It was awful. Part of me was heartbroken but another part was glad to know that he would have no more suffering'. In my experience, grief reactions are often prolonged, often into the pathological time. Partners who have cared for their adult child, who have never considered themselves carers (an acknowledged characteristic of this group of parents) and have never questioned why they should carry on are often left wondering what relationship they can now have together without the focus of their lives for the last 20 to 30 years. Mencap has literature for bereaved family carers and also for adults with intellectual disability if the carer dies first.

LEAVING HOME

Either because the carers realise that their old age is preventing them from offering adequate care, or because the young adult expresses a desire or need to gain independence or because the social or health advisers suggest it there comes a time when the young adult with intellectual disability moves to a communal home or residential care. Points to be considered are as follows.

➤ Who decides when the time has come for the young adult to leave home – the young adult or the family or others acting as advocates for the young adult to achieve more personal freedom?

➤ It is clear that when the family takes part in discussions about the placement the placement is more successful.

➤ The parents will have been subject to frequent and regular changes of local policy and may be doubtful about the success of any placement.

➤ When a placement in care is made discussion has to involve who is responsible for making decisions about the patient's medical care and giving consent in long-term care and in acute situations.

CARE AWAY FROM THE FAMILY

Residential or communal care for adults with intellectual disability is:

➤ owned and run by a local authority

➤ owned and run by private enterprise

➤ owned and run by the health service and rarely for patients with severe multiple disabilities.

Increasingly, the care is offered by private agencies on a commercial basis or under the conditions of charitable status.

The healthcare workers (support workers) caring for adults with intellectual disability come from varying backgrounds:

➤ the specialist practitioner – with specialist training in the field of social work or nursing

➤ the generic worker – with general training in social work or nursing

➤ the care worker – with no particular training other than that gained by personal experience in care.

Usually, each resident has a key worker who has particular knowledge of his/her care. An adult with intellectual disability usually consults with a carer and is essential for the GP or nurse to be aware of the experience and understanding of that carer.

SIBLINGS OF ADULTS WITH INTELLECTUAL DISABILITY

➤ Siblings of an adult with intellectual disability have had the relationship between them and their parents affected by the learning disability.

➤ Their own relationship with others such as school friends can be affected.

➤ They may not have learnt appropriate sibling relationships and this may make it difficult for them to form other relationships.

➤ They may have constant anxiety about feeling obliged to care for their intellectually disabled sibling if their shared parents die or become unwell. In general the parents are keen to make provisions for the adult with intellectual disability that do not place obligations on their other children.

➤ As they become middle-aged and their parents become frail they may feel they are more suited to supervising the care their sibling receives in care and this can lead to family conflict.

➤ If the adult with intellectual disability dies, they too will need specialised care in their bereavement.

➤ They may be intellectually disabled too if their sibling suffers mild or moderate intellectual disability.

FURTHER READING

• Department of Health (DH). *Family Matters: counting families in.* London: HMSO; 2001.
• Department of Health (DH). Adults with learning difficulties in England 2003/2004. Available at: www.dhgov.uk/en/Publications and statistics/
• Kerr M. Improving the general health of people with learning disabilities. *Adv Psych Treat.* 2004; **10**: 200–6.
• Lindsay PJ. 'Sunrise, Sunset' – transitions in the care of adults with learning disability. *Adv in Mental Health and Learning Disabilities.* 2008; **2**(3): 13–17.
• RCGP. *Supporting Carers: an action guide for general practitioners and their teams.* RCGP EKU Topic 4; 2009.
• Sutton E, Factor AR, Hawkins BA, Heller T, Seltzer GB, editors. *Older Adults with Developmental Disabilities: optimizing choice and change.* Baltimore, MD: Paul H Brookes Publishing; 1993.

CHAPTER 3

Common presentations

'John's behaviour has gone right off'.
'Jenny's not her usual self'.
'Bill isn't eating for some reason'.

These vague descriptions may resonate in an all-too-familiar manner for the busy general practitioner who cares for people with intellectual disability. The GP may be untrained in managing the health of people with intellectual disability and may be unfamiliar with the person or their carer – and the carer may have omitted to bring crucial information regarding past medical history and current medication. As a consequence the GP can understandably feel overwhelmed by the complexity of the situation and the challenges of making an assessment.

This chapter suggests an approach to some common presentations. It is designed to assist with preparing a short-term plan for helping the patient within the confines of a standard 10- to 15-minute general practice appointment. The chapter also encourages the establishment of a more thorough, holistic health assessment and coordinated plan in the longer term.

ASSESSMENT

People with intellectual disability suffer the same range of everyday illnesses as anyone else. Often, however, these conditions occur more commonly, due to the presence of physical impairments or the inability to communicate prodromal or initial symptoms. People with intellectual disability experience between two to four times the numbers of health problems compared to the general population. There are specific skills that will help GPs provide an effective assessment of people with intellectual disability (*see* Box 3.1).

BOX 3.1 Assessment tips for GPs: the six As

1 Assess communication skills and remember expressive skills do not reflect receptive skills.
2 Allow sufficient time and develop rapport.
3 Arrange adequate follow-up and collect information from multiple sources.

4 Adopt a bio-psychosocial approach.
5 Be aware of syndrome-specific conditions and the 'occults'.
6 Assume there is a cause of the health problem beyond the intellectual disability.

A thorough history and examination provide the basis on which to establish a diagnosis and commence management. Obtaining these details can involve challenges when dealing with the population with intellectual disability. A person with disability may not be able to verbalise pain, dysfunction or emotional distress. It is therefore particularly important that a carer who knows the person well, and genuinely has the patient's best interest at heart, is present to assist with the consultation process.

A brief history and examination may reveal obvious health issues to be addressed (e.g. a rash, blocked ears or a chest infection), but these may not be the reason for the initial call for help.

Depending on the nature of the presenting complaint and the urgency of the situation, a longer appointment can be scheduled in the days ahead. Encourage the carer to bring all available information about the person they are responsible for. *See* the checklist in Box 3.2 for particulars.

BOX 3.2 Checklist of patient details for use by the doctor and other clinicians

Patient details of primary importance:
● past and current medications
● allergies
● diet
● history of illnesses and operations
● family history
● person responsible for medical decisions.

And if they exist:
● a bowel care plan
● seizure charts
● behavioural records.

And also a personal history, including:
● family involvement
● favourite activities
● past residential information.

It may take a few appointments to achieve an adequate understanding of a complicated history, and to establish sufficient mutual trust to allow uncomfortable examination tasks or procedures (such as taking blood) to occur. It may be impossible to achieve compliance with some activities, even after a good deal of quiet explanation and coaxing, and unless it is likely to jeopardise their future health and well-being the person's right to refuse this must be respected.

If a different carer presents at later visits, it provides a chance to corroborate the history; often a completely different story can ensue.

SYMPTOMS MORE COMMON IN PEOPLE WITH DEVELOPMENTAL DISABILITY

The following are symptoms that present more commonly for people with intellectual disability:

➤ weight gain or loss
➤ halitosis
➤ pica
➤ gastric reflux and regurgitation
➤ cough and nasal discharge
➤ inability to cope with menstruation
➤ spasticity and contractures
➤ challenging behaviour.

Changes in weight

We all experience fluctuations of a few kilograms in bodyweight depending on the time of year, levels of stress, activity and motivation, and other lifestyle issues. More marked weight changes in the person with intellectual disability can be a vital clue to the presence of unheralded chronic illness, including malignancy. Often accompanied by changes in sleep patterns and behaviour, weight gain or loss can point to undiagnosed mental illness (such as depression or bipolar affective disorder), and prompt appropriate pharmacological intervention is necessary.

Clinical scenario

Martin is a 32-year-old man with intellectual disability of unknown cause. He has been institutionalised for most of his life. He speaks only a few words, but until two years ago was active and sociable, and able to carry out simple tasks. Over a period of several months Martin lost 12 kg, became very quiet and withdrawn, and seemed to lose the ability to feed and dress himself. Extensive medical examinations were carried out, with no positive findings. A malignancy was suspected but not proven. When it seemed that all physical causes for the changes had been excluded, Martin was referred to a psychiatrist and severe depression was diagnosed. He did not respond at all to several antidepressant medications used in increasingly high doses, so following appropriate consent from his institution and the state guardianship board, Martin was given a course of electroconvulsive therapy (ECT). The results were dramatic and over a period of several months he regained his previous skills and his former weight. He is now well managed with intermittent courses of ECT and small amounts of medication.

Pica, halitosis and nasal discharge

Atypical presentations are common in people with intellectual disability and usually require a detailed assessment and comprehensive investigations. Symptoms and signs, such as halitosis or nasal discharge, may have unusual causes and the diagnosis may be elusive. Pica behaviour is common in some people with intellectual disability and needs to be considered in the differential diagnoses.

Clinical scenario

Mark is a 46-year-old man with severe intellectual disability who enjoys good physical health. He has, however, a long history of pica with X-rays often demonstrating non-food items, especially small metallic objects. He presented with grossly unpleasant halitosis. On examination Mark appeared undistressed with normal observations, no local lymphadenopathy, some nasal congestion, no obvious dental caries or gum disease, and a slightly distended abdomen. His breath was fetid. Given his history, bowel obstruction secondary to pica was a possibility, but apart from a couple of paper clips, abdominal X-rays demonstrated no faecal overload and bowel gas patterns were normal. Dental review confirmed no causative pathology. A computerised tomography (CT) of Mark's sinuses, however, revealed congestion in his maxillary sinuses, and at review by an ear, nose and throat specialist several purulent pieces of polystyrene (possibly from a disposable cup) were removed from his nose, with subsequent resolution of his symptoms.

Reflux and regurgitation

Reflux disease may not be obvious.

The prevalence of gastro-oesophageal reflux disease is high in people with intellectual disability. The presence of GORD can be obvious, with symptoms ranging from gross regurgitation to belching after meals; however, reflux disease may not be evident. Acid suppressants, antiemetic drugs and cautious use of prokinetic agents can all assist symptoms. Surgical fundoplication is necessary in more severe cases.

More often, however, the presence of this condition is insidious with anorexia or subtle changes in behaviour (indicating discomfort) being the only symptoms evident. An unexplained cough, particularly at night, should warrant consideration of reflux or chronic sinus pathology.

Infection with *Helicobacter pylori* occurs much more commonly in people who live in institutions or group homes than other settings. Faecal antigen testing can be used to check for *H. pylori*. Faecal antigen tests can also be used to confirm eradication after treatment.

Clinical scenario

Maxine is a 44-year-old lady who has intellectual disability and spasticity of her lower limbs. She has lived in an institution for most of her life. She has no speech and limited non-verbal communication. Over a period of two years she developed an increasingly frequent pattern of putting her fingers down her throat, causing her to gag and have frequent small vomits. She was constantly grizzling and lost weight steadily until she was very thin.

Over a period of time Maxine was treated with antiemetics, antacids, H_2 inhibitors and proton pump inhibitors, all giving minimal or no improvement. Most of the staff working with her considered that she was exhibiting this behaviour to attract attention.

A psychologist and physiotherapist were called in to assist, and a behaviour management plan was instituted. Splints were applied to her arms, making it impossible for her to get her fingers in her mouth. She was commenced on antidepressant medication and given rewards for eating and not regurgitating.

When there was no improvement in her weight or mood, Maxine was referred for endoscopy, which demonstrated gross gastro-oesophageal reflux for which the only real treatment option was surgical fundoplication. The gastroenterologist recommended further trials of medication (in spite of a complete failure of medication previously) and expressed reluctance to recommend surgery on someone with such severe disability. Maxine's doctors advocated for the surgical option, and this was finally carried out. Three months after her surgery Maxine was eating well, gaining weight and no longer required arm splints or antidepressants. She is now starting to smile.

Inability to cope with menstruation

Some women with intellectual disability exhibit challenging behaviour during their menstruation; generally, they do not understand what is happening, and are confused and upset by it. They may express their displeasure and draw attention to their discomfort by smearing blood. They may be most reluctant to wear any sort of pad, especially if their achievement of faecal and urinary continence in childhood attracted much praise.

Clinical scenario

Helen is a 15-year-old girl with moderate to severe intellectual disability. She is non-verbal, but has reasonable receptive language. She arrived at the surgery with her mother who explained that Helen had just started menstruating and was not coping with her periods. She had been stripping off her clothes and smearing menstrual blood around her room and over her face. She would not tolerate pads or tampons. This had occurred in public, causing considerable embarrassment for her parents and younger sister. Helen's family were at a loss as to how to approach this situation.

During the consultation, Helen presented as a restless girl, unable to sit still. She was wearing jeans and a top, and was constantly trying to undo her jeans in an attempt to remove them. On examination she had no detectable abnormalities, including no sign of dysmenorrhoea. Her menstrual loss was moderate, but not excessive.

Spend time explaining menstruation to women with intellectual disability in terms that they can understand – using a book with simple illustrations can be helpful (see www.easyhealth.org). Dressing women in clothes that still look nice but are extremely difficult to remove (e.g. overalls with back fasteners) can be effective in controlling inappropriate behaviour, but it is extremely important to explain to the woman that these clothes are to help her to look attractive and make it easier for her to cope with her period, rather than being presented as a disciplinary measure. See also 'Menstrual management' in Chapter 21 (p. 170).

Spasticity and contractures

Spasticity can cause difficulties both for the person with the disability and for their support persons. Small improvements can make an enormous difference to the quality of life for people with spasticity.

Clinical scenario

John is a 52-year-old man with severe intellectual disability, who has a history of mild spasticity secondary to cerebral palsy. He used to be ambulant (albeit stiff-legged) and walked on his toes; however, gradually over the past two years his spasticity has increased to the extent that he is now bed-bound with severe flexor and adductor spasticity of his limbs. A CT scan of his head shows non-specific degenerative changes, while a thorough neurological review has found no other cause for his decline. His support persons became concerned about a small ulcer on his right chest wall where his right elbow had been fixed by his shoulder adductors, as well as red areas on the inside of his knees where they were pressing together. His left elbow crease was also very red and moist, and his support persons were unable to obtain elbow extension in order to clean and dress this.

Protective dressings were applied to John's areas of skin compromise where possible, and oral medication commenced. Diazepam proved too sedating, and baclofen (a peripherally acting agent) was ineffective. However, using the centrally acting drug dantrolene, a small amount of knee abduction was obtained, allowing the placement of soft wedges to separate his knees with consequent healing of the pressure sores.

John's right elbow remained fixed at his chest. Administration of intramuscular botulinum toxin to the right shoulder abductors produced enough muscle relaxation to allow separation of his elbow from his chest, and appropriate dressing and healing. His left elbow had progressed to the stage that tendon contractures predominated, hence agents acting on skeletal muscle were ineffective; surgical measures were required to prevent skin breakdown.

John's case illustrates an extreme example of how debilitating spasticity can be. Increased muscle tone and tendon contractures are very common in people with intellectual disability; they are generally undermanaged, and provide much discomfort and loss of function. Energy expended by spastic muscles can lead to weight loss. Management should be directed at relief of distress, minimisation of secondary pathology and optimisation of function, rather than necessarily achieving 'normal' ranges of movement.

Challenging behaviour

Behaviour is a method of communication.

Breakdown in communication between people with intellectual disability and their support persons and clinicians is a cause of much morbidity and mortality. Well-developed communications skills are essential to understanding a person's problem. Non-verbal communication is of crucial importance for the individual without speech, and behaviour is a powerful example of non-verbal communication. Further details are in Chapter 4, 'How to Communicate with your Patient' (p. 29).

For more information on challenging behaviour, *see also* Chapter12, 'Challenging Behaviour' (p. 93).

Consider physical causes of challenging behaviour

Any health problem can lead to pain and discomfort in a person with disability, and may present in an atypical manner. At initial presentation, there may be no clue to the underlying disorder.

Many physical conditions are more prevalent in people with intellectual disability. These include musculoskeletal or dental pain, unrecognised infections, constipation and bowel obstruction, and gastro-oesophageal reflux disease.

> **Clinical scenario**
>
> Terry is a 58-year-old man with moderate intellectual disability of unknown origin. He has autistic tendencies and has suffered epilepsy since early childhood, for which he is taking two antiepileptics. Terry does not speak but indicates some of his needs via gestures. He toilets himself, but is very private about this and immediately flushes the toilet after use.
>
> He presents with a three-week history of loss of appetite and has been noted to be banging his head more frequently than usual. He has also been yelling in his bedroom, which is uncharacteristic for him.

In considering possible causes of Terry's altered behaviour, it is evident that on the information given (which is often all the GP may receive), any of the above ailments could be responsible for his symptoms.

Dental conditions and reflux disease can cause pain associated with eating, and can subsequently lead to self-harm. Nausea and discomfort from a urinary tract infection, as well as otitis media, chronic sinusitis and constipation, can cause anorexia and precipitate or perpetuate behaviours that indicate distress. Long-term antiepileptic therapy and inactivity can predispose to osteoporosis. An undiagnosed fracture, or a joint or muscle injury, can cause discomfort and loss of appetite. Pneumonia can occur, even in the absence of cardinal symptoms such as cough.

The doctor must examine the patient thoroughly, and have both a high index of suspicion and a low threshold for investigations such as urinalysis, blood tests, X-rays and endoscopy (unless undue stress is likely to accompany them) to enable a diagnosis to be made and appropriate treatment instituted.

Consider environmental causes of challenging behaviour

Many people with intellectual disability have little control over their lives and they are very dependent on familiar faces and daily routines. For some, this is a hangover from the rigidity of institutional residency in long-term hospital; others (e.g. those with autism) have phenotypic characteristics that demand a predictable environment.

Unanticipated disruptions to the external environment can provoke significant emotional and psychological distress, and behaviour can be the only means of communicating this.

People with intellectual disability (as do those without disability) form close attachments to family and other support people. The loss of a long-term support person may be similar to the death of a family member, and can be met by a grief reaction that, unless anticipated, can be hard to recognise. Similarly, the cessation of a favourite activity or much anticipated routine can engender feelings of loss, which, in a non-verbal individual, may only be expressed by actions.

In assessing causes of altered behaviour, look at changes in staff or roommates at the residential home. (An individual with no disability who is roomed with someone they dislike, or forced to spend several hours a day in the company of someone who upsets them, is likely to express considerable dissatisfaction with the arrangement; there is no reason to expect people with developmental disability to be any different in this regard.)

Consider psychiatric causes of challenging behaviour

Psychiatric illnesses (which are more prevalent in people with intellectual disability) need to be considered along with physical and environmental causes of challenging behaviour.

FURTHER READING

- Durvasula S, Beange H. Health inequalities in people with intellectual disability: strategies for improvement. *Health Promot J Aust.* 2001; **11**(1): 27–31.
- Lennox NG, Diggens JN, Ugoni AM. The general practice care of people with intellectual disability: barriers and solutions. *J Intellect Disabil Res.* 1997; **41**(5): 380–90.
- van Schrojenstein Lantman-De Valk HM, Metsemakers JF, Haveman MJ, *et al.* Health problems in people with intellectual disability in general practice: a comparative study. *Fam Pract.* 2000; **17**(5): 405–7.

CHAPTER 4

How to communicate
with your patient

For good quality medical care to result, the doctor must take time establishing the best possible communication link with the person with intellectual disability.

Taking a history, assessing a patient, making a diagnosis, and determining a treatment or management plan all involve communication. It is the cornerstone on which rapport is established, and is used to convey information and instructions to the patient. However, people with intellectual disability often have major communication difficulties which are one of the most significant barriers to general practitioners providing high quality healthcare in this population.

IMPORTANT ISSUES IN COMMUNICATION

Research indicates that people with intellectual disability appreciate doctors who:
➤ talk to them respectfully
➤ do not shout
➤ explain what is happening
➤ treat them as if they are worthwhile
➤ listen to what they are trying to say
➤ say when they do not understand them
➤ allow enough time for a consultation.

Focus on abilities, not disabilities:
➤ Recognise and utilise the person's strengths – not weaknesses – and emphasise these in the consultation.
➤ Regard disabilities and impairments as problems to be circumvented, not the essence of the person.
➤ Assess capabilities by asking simple introductory questions (e.g. name, date of birth, reason for attendance).
➤ Involve the person through what they can do, e.g. 'Why not take your shirt off?' 'Thanks, that's great'. 'Show me on your communication board if you like'.

Establish rapport

Establishing rapport facilitates the communication of information, helps build sufficient trust and familiarity to proceed with the examination and investigations, and improves patient compliance. While obtaining information from the support

persons, establish rapport with the patient by maintaining as much contact as possible:
➤ Use verbal comments and affirmations, eye contact, facial responsiveness.
➤ Include the patient in explanations and plans.
➤ Show the patient examples (e.g. point to a model, tablets or other medication).
➤ Use appropriate physical contact.

Obtaining information from other sources

To obtain sufficient information to enable you to make a diagnosis and manage your patient's presenting problem, you will often need to seek information from other sources. This is especially the case where the patient has developmental disability with cognitive and communication problems.

Inform the patient that you would like to talk to someone else, or obtain reports from elsewhere – and you would like to obtain their consent for this. Even people with quite severe disability can often indicate that it is alright to talk to their accompanying people, and they may be able to nominate who they would like to speak on their behalf. Stress that the patient can enter the conversation at any time if there is something they want to say.

MAXIMISE COMMUNICATION
Reception and pre-appointment procedures

When making an appointment for new patients, establish reception and booking procedures that facilitate communication and history taking. The receptionist must:
➤ routinely ask all new patients to bring relevant health information to each appointment
➤ check whether the patient has any special requirements (e.g. interpreter, sensory problems)
➤ consider making a double booking to ensure adequate consultation time.
➤ try to put the appointment near the beginning of the surgery session to avoid prolonged waiting.

Health records maintenance

Health records of people with intellectual disability are frequently inadequate or incomplete, and paid support people are often unaware of past investigations or diagnoses which have significant impact on the person's ongoing health (e.g. undescended testes, diagnosis of oesophagitis). Make time to trace a patient's past history. Although it can be time-consuming, it is often vital to their care.

Consultation time and frequency

Consultations are likely to take more time than usual, in order to establish rapport, assess communication abilities, unravel complex histories, complete an adequate examination, and provide clear explanations and instructions.

It may be appropriate to:
➤ spend longer than usual on the consultation
➤ terminate the consultation incomplete, and arrange to resume at a further time
➤ use several consultations to complete a full assessment and examination, keeping individual consultations relatively short and manageable (to avoid being overwhelmed by the complexity of the issues)

➤ review the patient on a regular basis, in order to establish familiarity and confidence.

FACILITATE COMMUNICATION AND HISTORY TAKING
Greeting your patient
When greeting your patient the following steps facilitate communication.

➤ Greet the patient first (before the relative or other support person if they also come to the consultation).
➤ Use respectful terms (as for another person of a similar age).
➤ Obtain the patient's consent to address them by first name.
➤ Avoid treating the patient as a child or in patronising, over-familiar tones.
➤ Use the knowledge acquired of the patient's verbal skills to determine the next step.

Assessing communication skills
Patients with verbal skills

If the patient has verbal skills, ask them to introduce the other people accompanying them at the consultation; ask also about the role they play in the patient's life, e.g. 'Who do you have here with you today?'

Check that the patient is happy for any accompanying people to remain during the consultation. Indicate that they can ask anyone to leave at any time and state that you would like to spend some time alone with the patient if they are willing. Ask the patient what the presenting problem is.

Some people with mild intellectual disability have good expressive skills but poor receptive skills. They may give perfectly coherent answers to questions, but they may not understand the meaning. It can take some time before any inconsistencies become apparent.

Patients with limited verbal skills

If the patient has limited verbal skills, still address the patient. State that it is your intention to talk to the accompanying people about them – if that is alright, e.g. 'I'd like to find out more about you, Mr Brown, so I'll just ask your friends a few questions if you don't mind'.

Observe the nature of response to this and use it as a guide to decide the level and nature of further involvement with the patient.

Even if the patient is unable to understand spoken language, they may respond to the tone of voice or facial expressions; they can be included in the consultation in this way.

Sometimes an accompanying person acts as an interpreter of the patient's own communicative attempts, by explaining what signs or gestures mean, restating dysarthric speech or acting as a facilitator for facilitated communication (*see* Chapter 5, 'Methods of Communication', p. 34). Always look for concordance between what you are being told that the patient is saying, and your own assessment of what is being communicated (as judged by facial expression, sounds made, level of engagement and other non-verbal cues).

If uncertain of verbal skills

When uncertain about the patient's level of communication, initially assume competence – speak directly to the patient, and adjust as necessary, e.g. 'You seem a bit uncertain about answering my questions. Is there someone here who you'd like to help you with the answers?'

If a relative or other support person immediately assumes that communication will occur through them, e.g. 'John can't talk, doctor; he doesn't understand anything', be firm in first establishing contact with the patient, e.g. 'That's alright. I'd still like to talk to John to start with'.

Levels of receptive and expressive communication can sometimes be underestimated, even by relatives and other support persons who have known the patient for a long time. Be alert for indications that the patient is listening and following the conversation, and respond appropriately to this.

Using clear communication

There are certain techniques to adopt that assist in clear communication:
➤ Gain the patient's attention – and eye contact if possible – by using their name, or with touch. Do this before speaking.
➤ Use simple words, sentences and concepts.
➤ Avoid jargon; adopt age-appropriate terminology that is familiar to the patient.
➤ Use clear, direct, well-paced delivery, with concrete and obvious examples or figures of speech.
➤ Expect a response, and wait at least 10 seconds.
➤ Rephrase questions, if necessary.
➤ Supplement speech with body language (e.g. signs, gestures, facial expressions and demonstrations that use yourself or objects).

Using repetition

Repetition is helpful to reinforce a message and establish the importance of information. It also allows time for the patient to process the message. Having the patient restate what was said demonstrates whether the patient has understood. (Some people with developmental disability say they understand because they want to please you.)

Don't be afraid to tell the patient that you don't understand – never pretend to understand when you don't. Be honest and seek clarification, e.g. 'I'm not sure I quite followed what you said then. Can you tell me again?'

Asking open-ended questions and giving a choice of alternatives

Some people with intellectual disability will tend to say 'Yes' to direct or closed questions, e.g. 'Do you get the headache every day?' 'Yes'. If you suspect this is happening, you can subtly check, e.g. 'Do the headaches come only at weekends?' 'Yes'.

Preferably, use open-ended questions, e.g. 'How often do you get a headache?' However, some people with intellectual disability may find such questions overwhelming or conceptually difficult. A suitable compromise may be asking the patient to choose between two carefully selected alternatives, gradually narrowing the choice, e.g. 'Do you get headaches every day or sometimes? . . . Only sometimes?' If you suspect the answers are a parroting of the second alternative, rephrase and check.

Ask the patient to explain things back to you as often as is necessary to satisfy yourself that you are being understood, and that you understand what the patient is telling you.

Providing concrete examples and diagrams

Many people with intellectual disability have difficulty following abstract or conceptual language. Communication is enhanced by:

➤ using pictures (including anatomical references)
➤ showing simple diagrams or pictures (drawn yourself)
➤ demonstrating body parts and planned actions (on your own or a support person's body)
➤ allowing the patient to handle and explore the equipment
➤ modelling or acting out desired actions
➤ finding the appropriate picture or sign in the patient's communication book.

For information about alternative means of communications for people who have communication problems *see* Chapter 5, 'Methods of Communication' (p. 34).

Monitoring the patient's response

When talking to a support person, be aware of the patient's reaction to what is being said, and acknowledge it. Ascertain if the patient wants to be present during the discussion and is willing for the discussion to continue. Sometimes, a patient may choose to leave the room while uncomfortable topics are discussed.

If the information gathered from others present is sensitive or has upset the patient in any way, offer the patient the opportunity to talk to you alone about the matter.

In all situations where other people accompany patients in the consultation, offer the patient the opportunity to talk to you alone.

FURTHER READING

• Beukelman DR, Mirenda P. *Augmentative and Alternative Communication: management of severe communication disorders in children and adults.* 2nd ed. Baltimore: Paul H Brookes Publishing; 1998.
• Goode D. A *World Without Words: social construction of children born deaf and blind.* Philadelphia: Temple University Press; 1994.
• Musselwhite CR, St Louis KW. *Communication Programming for Persons with Severe Handicaps: vocal and augmentative strategies.* 2nd ed. Boston: College-Hill Press; 1988.
• Siegel-Causey E, Guess D. *Enhancing Nonsymbolic Communication Interactions among Learners with Severe Disabilities.* Baltimore: Paul H Brookes Publishing; 1989.
• van der Gaag A, Dormandy K. *Communication and Adults with Learning Disabilities.* London: Whurr Publishers Ltd; 1993.

CHAPTER 5

Methods of communication

People with intellectual disability have varied communication skills. People with moderate to severe levels of intellectual disability, for example, often are better at understanding than producing language.

People with poor language understanding (i.e. poor receptive language skills) rely on routines, and cues from their environments, to enable them to anticipate what will happen in a situation or to understand what someone is telling them.

Problems with language production (i.e. problems with expressive language) can result from not having the neuromuscular control to produce words. People with cerebral palsy, for example, may have good language skills but be unable to demonstrate them because of severe dysarthria. Similarly, some people with intellectual disability may be difficult to understand because of articulation problems; their attempts at spoken language are often unsuccessful, particularly with people who do not know them well. However, some people have severe language delays related to their cognitive impairment or to specific language deficits; their failure to speak or their use of only a few words is a result of problems with accessing vocabulary and formulating sentences, rather than with speech per se.

People who do not use speech, or whose speech is not functional in most daily situations, are said to have complex communication needs. These individuals use various forms of augmentative and alternative communication.

AUGMENTATIVE AND ALTERNATIVE COMMUNICATION

The umbrella term 'augmentative and alternative communication' (AAC) refers to:
➤ various informal and formal ways of communication
➤ techniques to access these communication modes
➤ strategies that people with complex communication needs can use to communicate.

The range of AAC systems is vast and encompasses both unaided and aided systems.

Unaided systems

Signs and gestures are considered unaided augmentative and alternative communication.

People with severe intellectual disability are likely to rely more on informal gestures, sometimes with a few formal signs, as well as informal means of communication that include facial expression and vocalisations, than other ways of communicating.

Gestures

Gestures can be made into a more formal system by having photographs of the person using the gesture, with a written explanation of the meaning in a communication book that accompanies the person, e.g. I rub my finger up and down my cheek when I need help.

A person can be taught new gestures within their skill repertoire to represent an expanding number of meanings. Gesture dictionaries can include other informal communication (such as facial expressions or behaviours) that are interpreted by family or other support persons to have a consistent and narrow range of meanings.

Key word signs

Many people with intellectual disability use key word signs taken from the Makaton vocabulary. Skills in using the signs will vary, from using a few basic signs to indicate wants and needs (e.g. food preferences, when help is needed, to stop an activity), to using a quite extensive vocabulary and producing simple two- to three-word sentences. Signs, used with people who can understand them, and in combination with other formal and informal systems, can be an effective means of quick communication.

Aided systems

Augmentative and alternative communication may incorporate the use of an aid. Aided systems can take many forms because they are usually designed according to the individual's needs and abilities. Aided systems vary according to whether they are non-technology-based or technology-based.

Non-technological systems

Non-technological systems include:
➤ communication boards and books
➤ charts with objects or pictures to represent a person's daily activities (e.g. a calendar)
➤ cards with written information that can be used by the person to access services in the community (e.g. a card to take to the hairdresser that says I'd like to make an appointment to have my hair cut)
➤ picture sequences that represent an activity or series of activities (e.g. attending a church service).

These systems employ symbols that the person selects to formulate a message. The symbols vary according to the language ability of the individual, but may include:
➤ the alphabet
➤ written words or phrases
➤ line drawings
➤ photographs
➤ objects, or parts of objects.

Technological systems

Technological systems include various electronic devices:

➤ simple message systems, in which a few messages are programmed under picture symbols, with a speech synthesiser speaking the selected message

➤ more advanced systems that allow combinations of symbols (e.g. the alphabet with picture symbols), the production of long messages with only a few selections, and integration with a computer to enable the person to move between oral communication and word processing or other computer activities.

Access techniques

Techniques for accessing aided systems include:

➤ directly touching a symbol, or pressing it with a fist or head pointer

➤ using a light pointer

➤ (with electronic devices) using a switch to activate the scanning of symbols, and pressing the switch again to select the desired symbol.

Another way is by using 'facilitated communication'. Facilitated communication is the term used when a person is physically supported by another person (a facilitator) in their use of a communication device. The correct use of this strategy involves a facilitator moving a person's hand back after a selection has been made to ensure the selection is clean (i.e. not influenced by the previous selection). Caution is needed when using this technique because of the potential for the facilitator to influence the content of the message.

With facilitated communication, the accuracy of the message cannot be assumed as the facilitator can unconsciously influence the content of the message. It is therefore important, when communicating with someone who is physically supported by a facilitator in the production of their messages, to be satisfied that the message is coming from the patient, by using other methods (e.g. body language, gestures, physical findings, yes/no or verbal responses, and opinions of other support persons).

MULTIMODAL COMMUNICATION

Augmentative and alternative communication is by its nature multimodal; it involves combinations of the methods outlined above. People who use signs, for example, will often also use a communication board or book, as well as their own gestures, vocalisations and facial expressions. The modality used may vary according to how familiar a person is with a communication partner, and the nature of the message they are trying to convey. A person who has a gestural dictionary as well as an extensive communication board, for example, is likely to use a gesture to communicate a quick message, such as 'Can you get me a coffee?' The person may then use the communication board to convey a detailed message about a recent incident.

Some individuals learn that unfamiliar people will not know their signs, and so will use a communication book with them, and signs for the same messages with familiar listeners.

COMMUNICATING WITH SOMEONE WHO HAS COMPLEX COMMUNICATION NEEDS

For people with complex communication needs, communication can be made less arduous if the listener spends time learning about how the person communicates and how the listener can assist in the communicating. People who use AAC are the best people to inform you of how to assist. This can be either through direct questions to the person using the AAC, or by observing the person communicate. Mostly, people who use AAC require patience from their listeners, and a willingness to work with them in the communication process.

Communicating with someone with complex communication needs who uses formal or informal AAC requires some simple but effective strategies.

Determining how the person communicates

Obtain as much information as you can about how the person communicates, with both familiar and unfamiliar listeners. Ask the support person to bring in any communication systems that the person has. Check the system to see if it contains any information on how the person communicates. (Many communication boards and books have a section for the listener describing how the person uses the system and any other informal modes of communication.)

If the person knows only a few signs, find out what they are. If unable to learn the signs prior to meeting with the person, ask the accompanying support person to interpret them for you (if they are used).

Sometimes, support people claim that a person does not have a communication system, or does not communicate. The latter is unlikely; instead the person probably relies on informal systems, such as facial expression or vocalisations. The person may also use inappropriate or problem behaviours to convey dislikes or express frustration due to being unable to communicate needs or wants; if this is suspected, intervention by a speech pathologist or an AAC specialist is warranted. If a person is reported not to have a communication system, ask the support person to tell you how he/she knows what the person wants.

Communicating directly to the person with disability

Some people have good communication skills but are only able to demonstrate them if attention is directed to themself rather than to the support person, and they are given plenty of time. If a person chooses to spell using an alphabet board or an electronic device, for example, ask if the person prefers that you anticipate the message (thereby saving the person the effort of completing it) or would rather that you wait until the message is completed. (People vary in their preferences; interruptions can disrupt a person's ability to process information.)

Even if you judge a person to have poor receptive language, still direct your communication to that person, rather than always directing it to the support person. Use simple but complete sentences. If the person has a communication aid, ask if it would help the person's understanding for you to use it for key concepts (e.g. pointing to a picture of a body part when asking if the person has pain there). Provide plenty of time for a response. Many people with intellectual disability require extra time to process information; for them, repeating information can be disruptive.

Consider using a series of direct questions that require a one- or two-word response. For people with good receptive language a series of yes/no questions can be used, but take care that people do not give the answer they think you want to hear.

Use your own AAC systems; these can take the form of pictures or gestures to help a person understand an explanation or instruction.

People who rely on routines will benefit from seeing a pictured representation of what will happen; they may also benefit from taking the picture home before returning for a procedure (such as a Papanicolaou [Pap] smear).

Communicating through a carer

If you find it difficult to understand a person's communication attempts, ask the person's permission to have the carer interpret or assist. When using this strategy:
➤ ensure you are getting a verbatim interpretation; stress that you want to know exactly what is said, even if it does not make sense to the interpreter
➤ allow extra consultation time for interpreting
➤ talk to, and maintain eye contact with, the person
➤ recheck and rephrase to clarify and enhance understanding of what the person is communicating.

FURTHER READING

- Beukelman DR, Mirenda P. *Augmentative and Alternative Communication: management of severe communication disorders in children and adults.* 2nd ed. Baltimore: Paul H Brookes Publishing; 1998.
- Duchan JF. Issues raised by facilitated communication for theorizing and research on autism. *J Speech Hear Res.* 1993; **36**(6): 1108–19.
- Ryan A, Keesing E, Cowley J. *The Makaton Vocabulary – Australian (AUSLAN) edition.* Australia: Makaton; 2001.

CHAPTER 6

Assessment of intellectual disability

Development, like growth, is something everyone does. Most developmental differences become apparent during early childhood and are assessed at that time. When a child seems to be developing differently from the expected, it raises the possibility that there may be something seriously wrong. While most children who present with concerns about development will have minor problems, it is always important to listen carefully to the parents' fears. Hasty or inappropriate reassurance may delay diagnosis and intervention, and undermine the parents' confidence in themselves and their doctors. Assessment should not ever be regarded as finished. New knowledge, new technologies and changing presentation dictate that the questions of diagnosis (in terms of both function and aetiology) need to be kept in mind throughout the life of the person with an existing or possible developmental disorder.

AETIOLOGY

Most developmental disabilities are due to factors that are operative before the onset of labour (i.e. preconception and during pregnancy) and result in differences in development (e.g. malformations of cortical development such as the neuronal migration disorders) and injuries to the developing brain (e.g. from infectious, toxic or hypoxic events). These can cause impairments in a range of neurological functions that affect the individual's ability to function in everyday life. Common disability categories include:

➤ motor functioning (e.g. cerebral palsy)
➤ cognitive functioning (e.g. intellectual disability)
➤ social functioning (e.g. autism spectrum disorders)
➤ sensory functioning (vision or hearing impairments).

Frequently more than one area of functioning is affected.

A developmental assessment should include aetiology – nominating the underlying cause – (e.g. Down syndrome, hypoxic injury) and functional impairment (e.g. intellectual disability, cerebral palsy). The rate of development also needs to be considered, as a small but important group of conditions are characterised by ongoing pathology and progressive functional deterioration.

Knowing the cause of the disability may:

➤ give information about when and why the disability occurred – important information for the person with the disability, their family and their healthcare providers to help them understand what has happened and aid grief management
➤ allow accurate assessment of risk to others, especially genetic risks to siblings and their families
➤ enable healthcare providers to access specific information relevant to the medical care (e.g. increased risk of thyroid dysfunction, depression and dementia in people with Down syndrome)
➤ enable families to locate information about the condition and find support groups.

A cause can be found for the disability in the majority of cases of moderate and severe intellectual disability (IQ<50), but less often in cerebral palsy, mild intellectual disability and autism. When a cause is identified, it is most likely to be a prenatal factor, approximately half of which are chromosomal abnormalities (particularly Down syndrome and fragile X syndrome). Table 6.1 gives some examples of the causes of developmental disability.

TABLE 6.1 Causes of intellectual disability

Category	Examples
Prenatal	
Genetic	Down syndrome, Angelman syndrome, Prader-Willi syndrome, fragile X syndrome, tuberous sclerosis, phenylketonuria, mucopolysaccharide storage disorders, some malformations of cortical development (e.g. lissencephaly, periventricular nodular heterotopia)
Acquired infection	Congenital rubella, toxoplasmosis, cytomegalovirus
Toxins	Foetal alcohol syndrome
Other	Iodine deficiency
Unknown	Dysmorphic syndromes (e.g. Cornelia de Lange), single malformation (e.g. microcephaly), multiple minor anomalies
Perinatal	Hypoxic-ischaemic encephalopathy, infection (e.g. meningitis, encephalitis)
Postnatal	Infection, trauma, hypoxia, poisoning.

PRESENTATION

The recognition of a disability in an adult may occur for the first time when the person presents to a medical practitioner because:
➤ of a change in their health
➤ a change in their behaviour is causing concern
➤ of an administrative or bureaucratic requirement
➤ of a change in accommodation.

Adults may also present because they or their carers feel that they have never been adequately understood or assessed.

Patterns of presentation

Walking, talking, self-caring, relating to other people, seeing, hearing and learning all require neurological skills; people with developmental disability may present with manifestations of delay in one or more of these areas.

Abnormal neurological development, whether due to brain injury or maldevelopment, frequently results in disturbances to more than one area of function. Disabilities therefore tend to coexist:

➤ autism frequently coexists with intellectual disability
➤ cerebral palsy frequently coexists with intellectual disability and/or a visual impairment.

Global developmental delay does not necessarily indicate widespread damage; but single impairments such as deafness, blindness and motor impairments tend to have global effects.

More than half of people with a developmental disability have one or more additional disabilities.

The pattern of presentation guides further investigation and management.

TABLE 6.2 Manifestations of developmental delay

Area of development affected	Manifestation	Possible neurodevelopmental diagnoses
Global	Delays in most areas	Intellectual disability, deafness, blindness, cerebral palsy
Motor	Late walking, motor delay, persistent primitive reflexes	Cerebral palsy, neuromuscular disorder
Language	Speech delay, limited understanding, unusual or inappropriate use of language	Specific language disorder, hearing impairment, autism, intellectual disability
Behaviour	Excessive colic or irritability, reduced or increased activity, aggression, sleep disturbance, odd or obsessive behaviour, narrow or unusual play patterns, interpersonal difficulties, social isolation, not fitting in	Autism, attention deficit hyperactivity disorder, intellectual disability, cerebral palsy

While ability patterns tend to be permanent, their presentation may change. Thus people may appear to have one type of disability pattern early in life and a different pattern as they become older. Ongoing review of the ability and disability patterns is therefore necessary.

History taking

The goals of history taking are:

➤ to define the nature and chronology of the developmental symptoms
➤ to explore the possibility of coexistent conditions (e.g. congenital abnormalities, sensory impairments)
➤ to identify the aetiology, where possible
➤ to identify factors in the individual, their family and the community that may influence the individual's development and prognosis (either positively or negatively).

It usually helps to talk with others who know the person in different settings; this may lead to a new understanding of the difficulties. Permission must be obtained for such conversations (which may be on the phone) – this is rarely a problem.

Examination

Listed below are important aspects of the examination of a person with an established or suspected intellectual disability.

Observation

Information about communication ability, behaviour and ability to interact socially with others in the room can be informally observed throughout the consultation.

General physical examination

General examination includes:
➤ measuring height, weight and head circumference
➤ taking note of dysmorphic features of the face, hands, feet and digits (see below)
➤ checking the ears, eyes (including visual acuity)
➤ examining heart and lung fields
➤ examining the abdomen (including pubertal development)
➤ examining neurological function
➤ assessing abnormalities of gait, limbs, and cranial nerves.

Dysmorphic features

Dysmorphic features need to be specifically looked for.
➤ Multiple minor congenital anomalies (i.e. those that do not affect function) suggest the presence of a major anomaly.
➤ Multiple minor anomalies in the presence of developmental delay suggest an intracranial malformation.
➤ Skin pigmentation abnormality may indicate abnormality elsewhere (e.g. tuberous sclerosis).

Investigations

The appropriate investigations depend on the findings of the history and examination. Investigations to be considered include:
➤ audiology assessment
➤ formal vision assessment
➤ karyotype testing
➤ specific tests for genetic disorders (e.g. DNA tests for fragile X syndrome, Angelman syndrome, Prader-Willi syndrome)

➤ electroencephalogram (EEG)
➤ brain imaging studies (e.g. magnetic resonance imaging [MRI])
➤ metabolic screening test
➤ other tests (e.g. creatinine kinase, thyroid function, phenylketonuria) as indicated.

If referral to a specialist is anticipated, it may be best to consider deferring the blood tests until the specialist visit; then blood for all tests can be taken at one time, avoiding undue distress.

FURTHER ASSESSMENT AND REFERRAL

When intellectual disability is suspected or identified, involvement of a specialist in the area may be appropriate. For children this is often a paediatrician; for adults the position is less clear. Suitable specialists may include neurologists, metabolic physicians, geneticists, rehabilitation physicians or designated disability management teams. These specialists can complete the developmental assessment and aetiological investigation, ensure contact with appropriate services and support groups, and monitor development over time.

TABLE 6.3 Contribution to assessment available from other professionals

Referral to	What the referral would provide
Geneticist	Information about aetiology and genetic implications and advice to siblings
Psychologist	Information about the level of intellectual functioning and areas of relative ability and difficulty
	Strategies for building skills
	Management of challenging behaviours
	Assistance to family members and carers
Speech therapist	Speech and language assessment and strategies to facilitate development of communication skills
Physiotherapist	Assessment of motor function and strategies to facilitate motor functioning
	Advice concerning appropriate aids and equipment
Occupational therapist	Assessment of fine motor and self-care skills
	Strategies to facilitate function in the fine motor and self-care areas
	Advice concerning appropriate aids and equipment

The GP needs to remain involved and informed about the individual's health and developmental issues over time, to ensure continuity and breadth of care. Good communication between the GP and others involved is central to good management.

Referral to a genetics service

Knowledge in the area of medical genetics has expanded rapidly over the last 10 years. Geneticists can provide assessment and advice on a wide range of genetic conditions, dysmorphic syndromes and currently available specific genetic tests. Genetic services provide genetic counselling for people wanting to understand their risk of having a child with a genetic difference, or wanting to decide how to proceed when such a diagnosis is suspected or known. Genetic services also provide public and professional education and are engaged in a range of research activities.

Developmental and psychological testing

Psychomotor development can be measured; standard tests are available. All areas of development (gross and fine motor skills, hearing and speech, self-help skills and social interaction) should be tested using standardised methods.

Tests are available for adults to quantify both general and specific developmental functions, e.g. the Wechsler Adult Intelligence Scale, 3rd edition (WAIS-III) and the Vineland Adaptive Behavior Scale.

Part Two

Routine care

CHAPTER 7

The adolescent with intellectual disability

Adolescence is a time of transition. Great physical and psychological changes occur as the young person develops a new social role. The relationship between GPs and adolescents should reflect this change – regardless of whether the adolescent has intellectual disability. This chapter provides an overview of medical, cognitive and social issues facing adolescents with intellectual disability and their families. Parents and families of adolescents frequently complain of the abyss of healthcare they encounter when their child with intellectual disability reaches adolescence – the overall, multidisciplinary team led, all embracing care of a community paediatrician gives way to fragmented care which must be promoted, developed and usually led, or more likely driven, by the GP.

ROLE OF THE GENERAL PRACTITIONER

Children with intellectual disability usually have a paediatrician who plays a central role in the coordination of their medical care. By late adolescence or early adult-hood, it is no longer appropriate for paediatric services to provide their healthcare.

In children with intellectual disability, ideally the GP and the paediatrician share a proactive holistic approach to the child's health and the family's well-being. There is, however, no equivalent to the paediatrician for adults with intellectual disability, and their healthcare becomes the province of the GP alone, with referral to specialist physicians and surgeons as appropriate.

The GP's active involvement during adolescence is important. As the transition to adult medical, educational and social services occurs, GPs can:

➤ ensure primary health needs are met
➤ offer ongoing health surveillance and coordinate specialist health services
➤ advocate for the family and assist with the paperwork required for service transitions
➤ support the child and their parents as they move from the often special and valued relationship with their paediatrician to new medical services
➤ nurture a trusting relationship with the young person during their teenage years, to facilitate the teenager becoming as active a participant as possible in their own health management.

The GP can encourage the individual and family to participate in a range of different relationships – with peers, friends, family and service providers – and to consider the different ways people can help and assist each other.

Many of the issues that arise for adolescents with disability (and their families) are the same as those arising for all adolescents in the community, and relate to the physical, emotional and social changes they experience. Tensions may arise between their own need for independence and autonomy, and their parents' need to protect and nurture them. Family therapy and cognitive behavioural therapy can be beneficial for some people in this situation. Physical and mental health issues may also lead to added complexities in management.

COMMUNICATION

One or both parents usually accompany a child with disability to medical consultations – and often speak for them. Gradually shifting the focus of the communication to the young person as they mature gives the message to both the young person and their parents that the consultation is now between the young person and their doctor, even if assistance is sometimes required. Communication with the adolescent is enhanced by:
➤ addressing the young person directly
➤ seeing the young person on their own for at least part of the consultation
➤ clearly stating the rules of confidentiality so the adolescent feels able to raise difficult or embarrassing issues.

MEDICAL ISSUES

Adolescents with intellectual disability have the same range of health concerns as their peers. There are, however, a number of issues that are particularly pertinent to this age group. These are summarised in Table 7.1, and some are discussed in more detail after the table.

TABLE 7.1 Checklist of issues to be addressed in adolescence

Issues to be addressed	Possible intervention
Health promotion and preventive measures	Provide education, advice and support on smoking and drug use, safe sex practices, contraception, health, diet, weight, exercise and fitness programmes Recommend standard immunisations as per the standard protocol as recommended in 'The Green Book' and encouraging hepatitis B, influenza and pneumococcal vaccine Referral as appropriate for specific support and counselling needs, e.g. drug and alcohol, human relations – often and usually under the administration of the Community Learning Disability Team
Mental health	Build resilience: focus on strategies to enable autonomy, independence, resourcefulness and achievement Identify risk factors and detect early signs of mental illness Interventions (e.g. cognitive behavioural therapy, family therapy) Refer to psychology or psychiatry services if indicated

Issues to be addressed	Possible intervention
Complex communication needs	Optimise independence and autonomy in communication Refer to speech pathology for communication assessment
Mobility	Optimise independent function Refer to physiotherapist for mobility devices (e.g. wheelchair) Refer to orthopaedic surgeon or rehabilitation physician for treatment of spasticity, or bone and joint disorders
Personal care	Provide education, advice and support on hygiene, continence and menstrual management as required Refer to disability worker, human relations counsellor or occupational therapist for skill development in personal care, including menstrual management if required
Sensory impairments	Regularly check for deterioration in vision or hearing Refer to audiologist or ophthalmologist if any concern or uncertainty
Endocrine dysfunction	Routinely check for endocrine dysfunction in conditions where increased risk is known (e.g. hypothyroidism/Down syndrome; precocious puberty/hydrocephalus; osteoporosis/non-weight bearing) Refer to endocrinologist if indicated
Epilepsy	Review seizure frequency, medication (type, dose, adverse effects, serum levels) as needed Address changes associated with puberty (i.e. seizure patterns may change in adolescence and medication dose will need to be adjusted as growth occurs) Refer to neurologist if indicated
Medication review	Regularly review medications; ensure rational prescribing including withdrawal of unnecessary medications
Social needs and services	Consider referral to: generic community services and disability services for social and leisure activities; social skills groups; support groups; accommodation, educational and employment services; case management

Pubertal changes

Pubertal changes in adolescents with intellectual disability usually occur at the same time and follow the same pattern as in their non-disabled peers. Disorders of puberty may be associated with particular conditions (*see* Table 7.2). If pubertal development does not fall within the expected parameters, consider investigations and referral for delayed or precocious puberty. Delayed puberty is associated with increased risk of cryptoorchidism which requires treatment in its own right.

TABLE 7. 2 Conditions associated with disorders of puberty

Pubertal disorder	Predisposing conditions
Precocious puberty	Hydrocephalus, intracranial tumours, microcephaly, porencephaly, post-infection (meningitis, encephalitis, toxoplasmosis), post-traumatic brain injury, tuberous sclerosis, hypothyroidism
Absent or delayed puberty	Prader-Willi syndrome, Klinefelter's syndrome, Turner's syndrome, Noonan syndrome
Small or ambiguous genitalia	Prader-Willi syndrome, Bardet-Biedl syndrome, Laurence-Moon syndrome, Klinefelter's syndrome, Down syndrome

Substance misuse

Drug use and abuse, including experimentation with tobacco and alcohol, may occur in adolescence and lead to potentially adverse consequences.

Tobacco use is a major health problem in people with mild intellectual disability; health promotion in this area is an important component of care.

Mental health

People with intellectual disability have an increased risk of developing mental illness throughout their life. There are many factors that increase the vulnerability of adolescents with disability to mental health problems. These include:

➤ **Biological factors** – people with differences in brain development and structure have an increased risk of both psychiatric illness and seizure disorders. Those with particular syndromes are at increased risk of specific mental illnesses (e.g. Down syndrome and depression, fragile X syndrome and social anxiety, Prader-Willi syndrome and psychotic illness).

➤ **Psychological factors** – cognitive impairments leading to a limited set of coping and social skills.

➤ **Social factors** – family factors (stress, lack of social supports) and community factors (limited social opportunities; lack of awareness and understanding; prejudice and discrimination).

Children with attention deficit hyperactivity disorder may become less hyperactive during adolescence, but the attention problems are likely to persist, requiring educational and behavioural interventions.

Adolescents with autism spectrum disorders have an increased risk of developing depression, anxiety disorders, behavioural difficulties and seizures.

Management

Address social risk factors, and support the adolescent to build their skills and resilience. The development of a strong sense of identity, robust self-esteem and resourcefulness can buffer against adversities encountered. This is assisted by:

➤ the presence of trusted relationships as sources of support and assistance

➤ the recognition of personal strengths and abilities by the individual and others

➤ opportunities to express and practise independence, autonomy and initiative

➤ circumstances in which the individual can achieve and exercise mastery and success.

Management of psychiatric problems follows the same principles that guide treatment of disturbed adolescents without intellectual disability.

➤ Assessment and intervention usually involve the family and/or other support persons, and school or workplace.

➤ Treatment usually requires the support and participation of support people (who may need to be educated in how to help).

The assessment and management of psychiatric problems in those with intellectual disability may require more time than in those without disability and a focus on building resilience and capacity, as well as addressing needs and vulnerabilities.

CARE OF THE FAMILY

The adolescent's family may also have needs to be addressed, including the need for:

➤ information on the physical changes of puberty and the implications for personal care and behaviour support – and services that could help

➤ information on the psychological changes of adolescence and the importance of balancing increasing autonomy with care and protection – and the services that could help

➤ practical assistance including financial assistance and respite care.

COGNITIVE ISSUES

Early childhood thinking processes tend to be concrete and involve the acquisition of literal facts. During adolescence cognitive abilities normally develop gradually to enable the manipulation of abstract ideas and the ability to organise and plan ahead.

Development in adolescents with intellectual disability

In adolescents with intellectual disability development of cognitive skills is delayed and/or impaired. Learning is slower, with the individual experiencing difficulties in abstracting and transferring learned skills into new settings. The ability to learn and develop continues throughout adult life (unless there is a degenerative or dementing process). Those working with people with intellectual disability should assist them to develop and make the best use of their individual skills and abilities.

PSYCHOSOCIAL ISSUES

The journey through adolescence involves a number of challenges, including:

➤ adjusting to changing physical and psychological states

➤ handling the changing expectations of others

➤ developing a sense of belonging to a peer group

➤ developing a sense of responsibility and reciprocity within relationships

➤ understanding and managing sexual feelings and needs

➤ developing a separate identity, value system and life direction from parents.

Each of these may present particular challenges for the adolescent with developmental disability.

Friendships

Identifying with a peer group is important to an adolescent's sense of well-being, self-esteem and to the establishment of their own identity (as distinct from their parents). Adolescents with intellectual disability may need more assistance and support in locating and participating in activities where friendships are likely to develop.

The development of trusting relationships, and an ability to identify and utilise sources of support and assistance, are important in building a sense of competence, autonomy, resilience and capacity in the young person.

Emergence of sexuality

An increased awareness and expression of sexuality during adolescence is part of normal maturation.

People with disability have the same sexual needs as others in the community, although the expression of their sexuality may be influenced by their social environment and their cognitive and social development.

Difficulty understanding the complexities of social relationships; limited opportunities to learn, develop and practise social skills with peers; lack of privacy; physical dependence on others; continence issues; loneliness, low self-esteem and encountering negative attitudes and low expectations of others may impede opportunities for normal sexual expression and hinder the formation of healthy sexual relationships.

Most teenagers acquire sexual knowledge from peers, the media and reading material. Poor literacy skills, restricted opportunities for adolescents with developmental disability to mix with peers and lack of knowledge within the peer group itself may all limit learning. School-based sex education programmes may not be tailored to the individual's level of knowledge, ability to process new information or cognitive level of understanding.

Inadequate knowledge, understanding and experience may lead to the adolescent expressing their sexual feelings in socially inappropriate ways. Specific information and targeted interventions may support the development of the knowledge, skills and behaviours required.

Intimate and sexual relationships (whether real or desired) become increasingly important to the young person as they mature socially and physically. Young men and women may need information and guidance in understanding the rights and responsibilities within relationships. GPs can have a significant role in sex education and in helping the individual and family adjust to the physical and psychological changes of adolescence. Referral to health and human relations counsellors may be helpful in some cases.

Increased independence from the family

It may be difficult for the family to adjust patterns of support to reflect the maturing adolescent and to assist them to develop an increasingly independent lifestyle. A family's reluctance to encourage the young person to develop interests, activities and friends outside the family may limit the adolescent's opportunities for independent experience. A certain level of supervision, protection and practical assistance may always be required; however, an increasing sense of independence in choice making and life autonomy are important in building resilience in us all.

Development of an adult identity

The development of individual identity involves an exploration of the ways in which the young person is separate from their family. Choice making, independent activities, testing of limits and abilities, belonging to a peer group and a sense of life direction are important components. Cognitive and physical impairments in the young person, and the parents' desire to protect them, can create barriers to the development of an adult identity and need careful consideration.

CHALLENGING BEHAVIOUR

In adolescence, some behavioural issues may resolve, while others may appear or worsen.

Adolescents with autism spectrum disorders and people with complex communication needs are particularly at risk of developing difficult or challenging behaviours.

Inappropriate behaviours can reflect a lack of knowledge, understanding or experience of social expectations.

Behaviours may also be a way of communicating feelings, needs or desires and a way of expressing physical or psychological pain and discomfort. Behaviours may be the symptom of a psychiatric illness or the demonstration of a behavioural phenotype. They may be a manifestation of seizure activity – or a way of expressing the frustration and desire for autonomy felt by many adolescents.

There are some factors that contribute to challenging behaviour that are particularly relevant to adolescence.

➤ Physical health: people with cognitive and communication impairments may have known and/or unrecognised medical conditions or experience adverse effects of medications that undermine their well-being and lead to behavioural changes.
➤ Epilepsy may arise for the first time in adolescence, and seizure types or patterns may change. Both auras and seizures can be associated with behavioural change.
➤ Mental health: people with intellectual disability have an increased risk of developing mental health issues.
➤ Psychosocial issues: behavioural difficulties may arise in those who have difficulty establishing an independent identity and lifestyle.
➤ Sexual and physical abuse of children with intellectual disability is more common than in the general population and the sequelae may include social, emotional and behavioural disturbance.
➤ Behavioural management strategies from childhood may lose effectiveness as the adolescent grows and develops physically and cognitively.

When challenging behaviour occurs, carefully evaluate the biological, psychological and social context of the behaviours.

When environmental factors are the cause of challenging behaviour modify the environment – do not use psychotropic medication.

Guidelines for the use of psychotropic medication to influence behaviour can be found in Chapter 13, 'Medication and Challenging Behaviour' (p. 103). There is, however, little research on the use of these medications in adolescents with intellectual disability and their use should be avoided if at all possible.

SCHOOL

Many adolescents with disability attend mainstream schools; others attend special schools or a combination of the two. Whatever the setting, it is the responsibility of the school to ensure the educational programme is designed to meet the student's learning needs. Depending on the student's individual educational requirements, this may include a combination of the academic curriculum and the teaching of functional life skills. Ensuring that the adolescent has a sense of belonging and being valued within the community, and is growing in their sense of competence and skill development, is a part of the educational plan for all children, including those with disability.

The school may require medical information or advice to better understand the adolescent's needs, to support them appropriately and to assist in the application for various entitlements.

The prospect of leaving school is a challenging one for any student. When a student has a disability both student and parents may be particularly apprehensive about the transition. The individual and the family may need support and help in exploring the range of post-school options available.

Transition from school

During the last years at school, transition arrangements to post-school alternatives will be discussed and planned for by a school staff member (e.g. the transition coordinator, integration teacher or welfare coordinator). Post-school options include open employment, supported employment, university, foundation courses, facility and community-based day centres, and individually tailored programmes. On leaving, coordination of service provision shifts from education to disability services.

Continuation of therapies

Many children with disability receive therapy services through school. The need for and access of ongoing therapy should be determined before leaving school. Options include generic services (such as community health centres) and disability specific services.

Medical reports may be required as part of the transition process in therapy provision.

Establishing new friendships

Leaving school can disrupt social networks. New friendships can be created at work, through special interest groups or shared activities. If the individual is unable to initiate or arrange these activities, a disability case manager may assist in identifying and organising appropriate social and recreational opportunities.

LEAVING HOME

During adolescence and early adulthood, some young people move out of the parental home. Disability services can assist in locating appropriate accommodation, although there may be very long waiting lists for supported accommodation. Families who feel their son or daughter may need this type of accommodation should investigate options well in advance to ensure they are included on an appropriate priority list.

FURTHER READING

- Australian Family Physician. Developmental disability. *Australian Family Physician*. 2004; **33**(8): 577–672. (Special journal issue on developmental disability)
- Blum RW. Improving transition for adolescents with special healthcare needs from pediatric to adult-centered health care (introduction). *Pediatrics*. 2002; **110**(6/2): 1301–3.
- Department of Health. *Family Matters: counting families in*. London: HMSO; 2001.
- Lindsay PJ. 'Sunrise, Sunset' – transitions in the care of adults with learning disability. *Adv in Mental Health and Learning Disabilities*. 2008; **2**(3): 13–17.
- Polzin U, Smith K. Integrating people with disabilities in the community. In: Annison J, Jenkinson J, Sparrow W, Bethune E, editors. *Disability: a guide for health professionals*. Sydney: Thomas Nelson; 1996.
- Scal P. Transition for youth with chronic conditions: primary care physicians' approaches. *Pediatrics*. 2002; **110**(6/2): 1315–21.

CHAPTER 8

Adult healthcare

Adults with intellectual disability experience the same range of healthcare problems as is commonly experienced in the general population; however, many of these problems occur with greater prevalence and remain unrecognised or poorly managed. In addition, adults with intellectual disability experience disorders that are associated with the aetiology of their disability.

The burden of illness may be increased in patients who cannot adequately communicate their symptoms as it may lead to failure of identification of the disease. This situation is made worse by other barriers such as negative attitudes of professionals and others; poor record keeping and follow-up by disability support staff; systems of support and healthcare that do not match the needs of the person.

Pain and infection are often unrecognised in people with disability and may present as a change in behaviour (e.g. tearfulness, withdrawal, aggression, increased irritability); these behavioural disturbances may be the only indication that a person is experiencing discomfort and may be perceived by support persons and doctors as the primary problem, while the underlying medical disorder remains unnoticed.

It is common that the cause of an adult's disability has been investigated in childhood; however, if the cause remains unknown, a review by a clinical geneticist should be undertaken. This review may assist in ongoing medical care of the adult. Until there is a definitive diagnosis, further review should occur every five years as genetics knowledge multiplies.

COMMONLY UNRECOGNISED OR UNTREATED CONDITIONS

Conditions commonly unrecognised or untreated in adults with intellectual disability include:

➤ mental health disorders (*see* Chapter 14, 'Assessment of Psychiatric Disorders', p. 111 and Chapter 15, 'Management of Psychiatric Disorders', p. 121
➤ visual impairments
➤ hearing impairments
➤ tooth and gum disease (*see* Chapter 19, 'Oral Health', p. 160)
➤ gastrointestinal problems – particularly severe constipation (especially in people with cerebral palsy), intestinal obstruction, *Helicobacter pylori* infection, gastro-oesophageal reflux disease, dysphagia

➤ musculoskeletal and joint problems – including unrecognised fractures and secondary discomfort

➤ chest infections – especially in people who are immobilised or at risk of aspiration (e.g. cerebral palsy)

➤ endocrine disorders – osteoporosis, osteomalacia, diabetes and thyroid disease

➤ poor nutrition – obesity and under-nutrition

➤ skin disease – such as acne and tinea.

Adverse drug effects occur more commonly in people with intellectual disability, and both health promotion and disease prevention are overlooked.

It is important for the GP to:

➤ ask about recent changes in behaviour

➤ perform a yearly comprehensive health review

➤ encourage six-monthly dental reviews.

VISION AND HEARING IMPAIRMENTS AND DISORDERS

People with intellectual disability experience a much higher prevalence of hearing and visual impairments, and eye and ear disorders, than does the general population. Studies of community populations of people with intellectual disability have found that up to 50% of people have unrecognised or inadequately managed visual or hearing impairments, and 5% have both sensory impairments.

Patients may not be aware of their sensory impairments or may be unable to communicate their problems. Carers often do not suspect or realise when a problem exists.

Hearing tests such as the whisper test at 3 metres, and vision testing using Snellen or picture charts, can be performed accurately on people with mild (and many people with moderate) intellectual disability. These tests are often not feasible in people with more severe disability, who should be sent to an audiologist and ophthalmologist/optician for regular review.

It is important to check correct use of hearing aids and glasses, while ensuring that adequate lighting, sufficient contrast and quiet environments are available to those with sensory impairment when they are communicating.

All people with intellectual disability who have vision and hearing impairment – even those with very severe disability – can benefit from an improvement in their sight and hearing.

If the provision of spectacles or hearing aids is not practical, support persons may change the environment in ways that improve perception and comprehension. Examples of environmental change include:

➤ turning off radios and televisions when speaking to the person

➤ speaking clearly

➤ removing glare

➤ increasing light

➤ providing contrast.

It is important for the GP to:

➤ perform an otoscopy yearly (especially for wax build-up in people with hearing aids)

➤ check correct use of hearing aids or glasses
➤ screen hearing and sight every three to five years using a whisper test at 3 metres and Snellen or picture charts (when the tests are inconclusive or are unable to be accurately performed, then regular screenings by an audiologist and ophthalmologist are necessary)
➤ use loupe devices in the surgery and consultation for patients with hearing aids.

GASTROINTESTINAL PROBLEMS
Gastro-oesophageal reflux disease

Gastro-oesophageal reflux disease occurs commonly in people with intellectual disability; it is most prevalent in people who have scoliosis, cerebral palsy, Down syndrome, an IQ<35, and in those who take antiepileptics or benzodiazepines.

Patients with intellectual disability often experience severe GORD and, as they may be unable to communicate their symptoms, clinicians need a high index of suspicion. It should be considered in cases of:
➤ challenging behaviour
➤ recurrent vomiting and aspiration
➤ anaemia or overt gastro-oesophageal bleeding
➤ poor growth and nutrition in children with cerebral palsy
➤ dental erosions
➤ self-injurious behaviour and frequent episodes of screaming.

For patients without alarm symptoms, a trial of therapy for a few weeks is warranted, and if effective should be continued. In the presence of alarm symptoms (such as pain on swallowing, dysphagia, weight loss or anaemia) endoscopy should be performed. Complications of GORD – including oesophageal ulceration, oesophageal stricture, Barrett's oesophagus and oesophageal cancer – often occur. Treatment should be tailored according to the severity of the disease.

Mild, intermittent gastro-oesophageal reflux disease

Most people with intellectual disability who have mild, intermittent GORD require regular treatment. However, for very intermittent or occasional symptoms, avoiding precipitating foods may be all that is needed. Other non-drug measures (such as elevation of the bedhead, avoidance of eating or drinking at bedtime, advice about weight reduction – if overweight or obese) and other lifestyle modifications (such as stopping smoking) probably have some benefit. Nonsteroidal anti-inflammatory drugs (NSAIDs) should be discontinued if possible.

If drug treatment is required antacid/alginate preparations, H_2-receptor antagonists and proton pump inhibitors need to be considered.

Gastro-oesophageal reflux disease requiring regular therapy

For patients who have gastro-oesophageal reflux symptoms on most days, ongoing treatment is usually indicated. The objectives are to relieve symptoms, heal oesophagitis (if present), and reduce the risk of developing complications. Proton pump inhibitors initially at usual dosage are essential.

If symptom response is inadequate, especially after treatment for at least eight weeks, or if the patient originally presented with a complication of the oesophagitis (such as bleeding or stricture), dosage may be doubled. There is evidence that higher-dose proton pump inhibitor (PPI) therapy is more effective when given twice daily rather than once daily.

Maintenance therapy

The longer-term aims are (in order of importance) to control symptoms (even if the symptoms cannot be verbalised), reduce the risk of developing complications and minimise long-term economic costs.

In most patients who are able to communicate symptoms, a trial of reducing the intensity of treatment is worthwhile, while monitoring the response according to symptom control (endoscopy is not needed). The exception is patients who were originally shown at endoscopy to have severe oesophagitis (as often found in people with intellectual disability), as these patients all relapse unless treated with daily PPIs. Others who require ongoing full- or double-dose PPI therapy are those with Barrett's oesophagus, strictures or scleroderma. Barrett's oesophagus and oesophageal cancer are both prevalent in people with developmental disability.

Antireflux surgery may be undertaken in some otherwise fit patients to avoid the need for long-term medication, or if there is poor symptom control with PPI therapy.

Helicobacter pylori infection

Helicobacter pylori infection is increased in people with intellectual disability who live or have ever lived in residential care (including institutions, group homes and respite care centres), and in people attending day centres. Of those who are chronically infected, *H. pylori* is associated with gastritis in 100%, peptic ulcer in 6% to 20% and gastric cancer in about 1%; it should therefore be screened for in individuals who are unable to complain of dyspepsia.

Diagnosis is possible using faecal antigen tests.

Individuals who are infected need eradication therapy as for the general population, usually with a proton pump inhibitor and amoxicillin and clarithromycin.

Constipation

Due to the common occurrence of constipation, it is often overlooked by the doctor, and not mentioned by the patient or support person during a consultation. However, constipation can be a cause of distress, and in people with intellectual disability the discomfort of constipation may cause challenging behaviour. Severe chronic constipation may result in recurrent hospitalisation, intestinal obstruction, volvulus and ultimately death. Constipation merits vigorous investigation and treatment.

The risk factors for constipation in people with developmental disability include:
➤ poor food and/or fluid intake, particularly in people with dysphagia
➤ poor mobility (e.g. those with significant physical disability)
➤ severe intellectual disability
➤ those with a low fibre diet, usually in conjunction with a diet high in refined and processed foods
➤ some medications.

Antipsychotics (which can cause constipation) are commonly used in people with developmental disability. Review the indications for all drugs that may cause constipation, including:

➤ drugs with anticholinergic properties – typical antipsychotics, tricyclic antidepressants, antispasmodics, antiparkinsonians
➤ atypical antipsychotics (risperidone, olanzapine, clozapine, quetiapine)
➤ aluminium- or calcium-containing antacids
➤ iron preparations
➤ opioids
➤ verapamil.

Management

The management of constipation is important as inadequate management can lead to faecal impaction, which causes urinary and faecal overflow. Preventive management consists of:
➤ a regular intake of dietary fibre
➤ engaging in physical activity
➤ the consumption of 1000 to 1500 mL of fluid per day (for children), and 1500 to 2000 mL of fluid per day for adults (insensible fluid loss from lungs and skin can be as high as 800 to 1000 mL).

Fluids may be taken in the form of water, drinks and liquid foods, and as a constituent of foods.

Once adequate fluid intake is established dietary fibre may be increased. The recommended amount of dietary fibre is 30 g per day, which should be introduced into the diet gradually to avoid adverse effects (such as bloating or flatulence). Patients should be encouraged to choose from a wide variety of fibre sources (e.g. wholegrain or wholemeal products such as breads, cereals, pastas and rice; fruits and vegetables; legumes; seeds and nuts) rather than adding a few very high-fibre foods (such as unprocessed bran) to the diet.

For a patient with dysphagia, it may be helpful to ask for a dietician's assessment of fluid intake and for recommendations on how best to increase fluid and dietary fibre intake. Also, a speech pathologist can advise on the most suitable texture of fluids and optimal methods of administration. Many people with dysphagia have difficulty taking sufficient food and fluids and may require the texture to be modified (e.g. thickened fluids, purees). They may also be dependent on a family member or other support person for timely provision and assistance with their eating and drinking. It is therefore important to give support persons detailed instructions on the amount of fluid required per day, and methods of administration.

Where dietary and exercise measures are ineffective, intermittent or regular use of laxatives may be necessary. The duration of treatment with laxatives should be limited to the shortest time possible; however, some people require ongoing use of laxatives to maintain an acceptable bowel habit.

Prolonged use of stimulant laxatives may occasionally result in an atonic bowel, perhaps because of damage to the myenteric plexus. Laxatives may also cause hypokalaemia.

Herbal preparations that may contain stimulants such as senna and cascara may also be taken.

FIRST-LINE THERAPY

If dietary management is not sufficient, bulk-forming agents, such as psyllium and ispaghula powder or granules, once or twice daily, are the laxatives of choice for mildly constipated individuals. Provided good fluid intake is maintained, use ispaghula bulk-forming agents, orally according to manufacturer's instructions.

The effect of bulk-forming laxatives is usually apparent within 24 hours, but two to three days of medication may be required to achieve the full effect.

SECOND-LINE THERAPY

Bulk-forming agents are not always effective, even for mild constipation; if the first-line therapy fails, use an osmotic laxative such as: macrogol 3350 powder, 1 to 3 sachets daily.

THIRD-LINE THERAPY

If constipation is resistant to the above measures, there should be a re-evaluation of the underlying causes (including impaction). For further therapy use a stimulant laxative.

FOURTH-LINE THERAPY

In a small number of people with developmental disability these measures may be unsuccessful and repeated enemas, macrogol 3350, sodium phosphates or sodium picosulfate bowel preparations and/or manual evacuation may be required (sometimes after admission to hospital).

URINARY INCONTINENCE

Primary incontinence (i.e. where continence has never been attained) is most likely a consequence of the person's disability (neurogenic and/or cognitive). Secondary incontinence and worsening of primary incontinence are usually the result of a factor other than the disability.

All cases of incontinence should be carefully evaluated to elucidate the cause and possible contributory factors.

The following questions should be answered:
➤ Is the incontinence primary or secondary?
➤ What are the lower urinary tract and bowel symptoms?
➤ What provocative factors are there?
➤ Are there any issues specific to the developmental disability, such as communication of needs, access to and security at the toilet, and other needs that have not been met (e.g. distress)?

Examination should include an abdominal, rectal, pelvic (in females), neurological and orthopaedic examination, as well as an assessment of general mobility and dexterity. A urinalysis should be done and a urinary diary (charting frequency and volume) may be helpful.

Investigations are influenced by the clinical situation, but may include urine microscopy and culture, urine cytology, urea, creatinine and glucose levels, urinary tract ultrasound, lumbosacral spine X-ray, cystoscopy and urodynamics.

Interventions should be tailored to the individual's needs and abilities, and may include:

➤ education of the individual and their support persons
➤ behavioural strategies
➤ treatment specific for the type of lower urinary tract dysfunction (e.g. anticholinergics and/or bladder training for detrusor instability, surgery for genuine stress incontinence, prostate-specific treatment)
➤ use of appropriate aids and appliances.

Referral for assessment and advice to a continence physician (usually a geriatrician – irrespective of the age of the individual), continence nurse advisor, urologist or urogynaecologist may be appropriate.

ENDOCRINE DISEASE
Osteoporosis
Osteoporosis is defined as bone mass density 2.5 standard deviations or more below the mean for young normal subjects. There is increasing evidence of high levels of osteoporosis in people with intellectual disability. The reported prevalence of osteoporosis varies according to the population studied, but one study of community-dwelling adults aged between 40 and 60 years found that 21% had osteoporosis and 34% had osteopenia.

The screening threshold for osteoporosis in people with intellectual disability should be lower than in the general population. A baseline bone mineral density (BMD) measurement should possibly be done in all people with intellectual disability; the result would guide future measurements.

Prevention
RISK FACTORS
The risk of osteoporosis increases with increasing age. Other risk factors include:
➤ small body weight
➤ impaired weight bearing
➤ impaired mobility
➤ impaired nutritional intake.

People with intellectual disability are more likely than others to have impaired weight bearing and impaired mobility. Other specific factors that increase the risk of osteoporosis and that are more common in adults with intellectual disability include:
➤ a diet low in calcium
➤ lack of vitamin D
➤ several drugs (including phenytoin and sodium valproate)
➤ delayed puberty
➤ amenorrhoea
➤ hypogonadism
➤ hypothyroidism
➤ Down syndrome.

VITAMIN D
People with intellectual disability who do not have regular skin exposure to sunlight should have serum 25-hydroxy vitamin D levels monitored annually (at the end

of winter when it is at its lowest) as they will develop vitamin D deficiency over a period of months or years. Only about 10% of the body's requirement for vitamin D can be obtained from the diet, even if foods high in vitamin D (such as milk, margarine, butter and oily fish) are regularly included. Measures to increase vitamin D levels include improving sunlight exposure and giving a vitamin D supplement (e.g. ergocalciferol 1000 international units daily). Some experts suggest routine supplementation with Vitamin D (e.g. ergocalciferol 400 international units daily is required). Vitamin D status may also be impaired in people receiving phenytoin.

CALCIUM
Adequate calcium intake is important. The recommended dietary intake (RDI) of calcium for adult men and women 19 to 54 years of age is 800 to 1000 mg per day; it is higher (1000 to 1500 mg) for pregnant women, adolescents and elderly women. The following are good sources of calcium:
➤ 1 cup (250 mL) of whole or skim milk – provides 290 mg calcium.
➤ Fat-reduced milks – are usually enriched with skim milk powder and contain more calcium.
➤ 1 slice (30 g) of natural cheddar cheese – provides 235 mg calcium.
➤ Yoghurt – has equivalent calcium as milk.

Sometimes milk and milk products are eliminated from a person's diet in the common (but mistaken) belief that milk causes excess salivary mucous and thus contributes to aspiration. Eliminating milk from the diet may compromise calcium intake and exacerbate bone demineralisation.

Serum calcium should be checked; however, levels will not necessarily provide a measure of true calcium status since there is a homeostatic mechanism to maintain serum calcium.

OTHER PREVENTION STRATEGIES
Where possible, physical activity should also be encouraged.

Management
Management measures include:
➤ excluding or treating underlying diseases (e.g. coeliac disease in Down syndrome, hypogonadism in men)
➤ measuring the severity of osteoporosis by BMD measurement – any patient who has sustained a low-trauma fracture especially needs BMD measurement. (Transmission ultrasound of bone is also available but a normal result does not rule out osteoporosis.)
➤ arranging appropriate therapy (such as calcium, vitamin D, hormone replacement therapy, bisphosphonates)
➤ removing risk factors for fractures
➤ treating pain
➤ restoring mobility.

Treatment for osteoporosis is not proven in people with intellectual disability and may not have the same efficacy. For example, if there is a specific osteoporotic problem in an individual with Down syndrome, it may not respond to therapy in the same way as in the general population; likewise the absence of weight bearing, such as in a person in a wheelchair or in those who are bedbound, may inhibit a therapeutic response.

Falls prevention

Patients with intellectual disability are unlikely to complain of the symptoms of osteoporosis, and the signs and symptoms of fractures may be missed. As people with intellectual disability are more likely than others to fall, with a consequent fracture, falls prevention is important. The morbidity associated with a fracture in people with intellectual disability is greater than in others.

Some measures to prevent falls are:
➤ improving vision (where practicable)
➤ improving household lighting and contrast, and eliminate glare
➤ reviewing medications (especially sedatives, and drugs altering gait or causing hypotension)
➤ providing necessary equipment to the residence (such as rails, modified toilet and walking aids) after a home safety assessment to modify environmental hazards. A qualified therapist – usually an occupational therapist – most often does this.

The risk of fractures can be reduced by providing hip protectors and involving patients in exercise programmes.

Osteomalacia

Osteomalacia (termed 'rickets' in children) is a common cause of bone fragility in people with intellectual disability. In adults, defective mineralisation of bone causes osteomalacia; in children, defective mineralisation of the cartilage in the epiphyseal growth plate causes permanent bone deformities – rickets. Osteomalacia in adults may result in osteopenia. Osteomalacia and rickets are usually caused by vitamin D deficiency due to:
➤ inadequate sunshine exposure
➤ inadequate diet
➤ some antiepileptic drugs
➤ fat malabsorption (e.g. coeliac disease).

Laboratory findings include low serum 25-hydroxy vitamin D, low or low-normal serum calcium and phosphate, normal or elevated alkaline phosphatase, normal or elevated parathyroid hormone. Radiographic findings of epiphyseal growth-plate abnormalities, osteopenia, cortical thinning and Looser's pseudofractures may be seen. The diagnosis is usually reached without recourse to a bone biopsy (although this is definitive and constitutes the gold standard for diagnosis).

Individuals who mainly live indoors, and those being treated for epilepsy, require regular screening for vitamin D deficiency. 25-hydroxy vitamin D should be measured annually at the end of winter. Supplement with vitamin D for as long as required, continuously if the risk is ongoing.

Thyroid disease

Thyroid disease can occur at any age and is especially common in people with Down syndrome and some other genetic diseases.

Hypothyroidism is the usual manifestation and may be either primary (due to thyroid failure) or secondary (due to pituitary or hypothalamic disorders). Secondary hypothyroidism may be accompanied by secondary hypogonadism, and needs specialist referral. Screening should occur yearly in people with Down syndrome and others at risk.

Hypothyroidism in people with developmental disability is treated with thyroxine and treatment is usually lifelong. Introduction of thyroxine must be done with care. Starting at a low dose and titrating only every six weeks is recommended. Monitoring for arrhythmias (especially atrial fibrillation), congestive heart failure and other complications of thyroxine treatment is important.

Hyperthyroidism may present as behavioural disturbance and weight loss. Specialist referral should be considered.

Diabetes

The prevalence of diabetes in people with intellectual disability is unknown, but in view of the increased obesity and inactivity in this population it is probably more common, and may be under-diagnosed. Diabetes is common in specific conditions, such as Prader-Willi syndrome where its control is difficult.

People with diabetes that require insulin may need specialist referral.

Respiratory disease

Respiratory disease is the most common cause of death in people with intellectual disability. Respiratory disease is often the result of chronic dysphagia leading to aspiration; it may subsequently present as recurrent respiratory tract infections or be misdiagnosed as asthma. A history of cough while eating or drinking should raise the suspicion of aspiration.

Aspiration pneumonia and lung abscess should be treated with high-dose oral antibiotics.

Asthma requires the same treatment as in the general population, but the patient may not be capable of the degree of self-management required by an asthma plan.

Sleep apnoea is common in obese patients and if weight loss or surgical procedures (such as tonsillectomy) are ineffective, continuous positive airways pressure (CPAP) may be necessary.

Chronic obstructive pulmonary disease (COPD) is less common because of the decreased incidence of smoking and should be managed along conventional lines, but there should always be a doubt about the diagnosis unless a cause can be identified.

For more information on aspiration and dysphagia *see* Chapter 18, 'Dysphagia' (p. 154).

FURTHER READING

- Beange H, McElduff A, Baker W. Medical disorders of adults with mental retardation: a population study. *Am J Ment Retard.* 1995; **99**(6): 595–604.
- Bohmer CJM, Klinkenberg-Knol EC, Niezen-De Boer MC. Prevalence, diagnosis and treatment of gastro-oesophageal reflux disease in institutionalised persons with an intellectual disability. *J Intellect Dev Disabil.* 2002; **27**(2): 92–105.
- Center J, Beange H, McElduff A. People with mental retardation have an increased prevalence of osteoporosis: a population study. *Am J Ment Retard.* 1998; **103**(1): 19–28.

- Draheim CC. Cardiovascular disease prevalence and risk factors of persons with mental retardation. *Ment Retard Dev Disabil Res Rev.* 2006; **12**(1): 3–12.
- Wallace RA, Webb PM, Schluter PJ. Environmental, medical, behavioural and disability factors associated with Helicobacter pylori infection in adults with intellectual disability. *J Intellect Disabil Res.* 2002; **46**(1): 51–60.

CHAPTER 9

Aged care

In the 1930s the average life expectancy of people with intellectual disability was around 20 years. By 2002, it had risen but still remains lower than general life expectancy – five years lower for those with mild intellectual disability and 20 years lower for those with severe intellectual disability. People with intellectual disability are 58 times more likely than the general population to die before the age of 50 years, with respiratory failure being the most common recorded cause of death. Premature death is associated with:

➤ increasing severity of intellectual disability
➤ general markers of physical disability and debility
➤ epilepsy
➤ cerebral palsy
➤ Down syndrome.

However, increasing numbers of people with intellectual disability, especially women, are now living into old age. The survivor population, who have mild intellectual disability, fewer comorbid conditions and high levels of adaptive functioning, have a life expectancy approaching – and in some cases exceeding – the life expectancy of the general population.

Great gains have also been made in the life expectancy of people with Down syndrome. The median age of death of a person with Down syndrome in the United States was only 25 years in 1983, but this doubled to 49 years by 1997.

The absolute numbers of older people with intellectual disability are small. The size of this older group is expected to double in the next two decades due to a combination of increasing life expectancy and the ageing of the baby boom generation.

GENERAL CLINICAL ASSESSMENT

Many health management issues are the same for all individuals who are ageing. However, clinical management of ageing adults with intellectual disability is often complicated. Family members are often unaware of changes that occur during the ageing process, and may attribute problems to the disability or behaviour, rather than to a change in health status secondary to ageing. Support people who are not family members may have a limited understanding of ageing, as they are often young and untrained; also they may have limited knowledge of the individual for whom they are caring. Older adults with intellectual disability may have frequent changes of support people and residential location, and health records are often inadequate. Consequently, it may take some time to piece together an accurate picture of the individual's health status.

A comprehensive approach to clinical assessment of those with intellectual disability requires more thought and time as the patient ages. Physical and psychological problems impact upon functioning and as age-related disability is added to the underlying problems of those with intellectual disability, functional and social aspects of the assessment become more important. Clinical information needs to be gleaned from several sources including family members, friends and formal support persons. Hearing and vision impairments are more common with older age. Attention to both face-to-face positioning while speaking and good lighting improves the quality of verbal communication.

Physical examination should be completed with particular attention to the cardiovascular, neurological and musculoskeletal systems. Functional status (particularly changes in ability to self-care) should be assessed routinely; social and financial needs should also be established.

Frailty is an important concept that applies to older people with intellectual disability. It can be regarded as 'a condition or syndrome that results from a multisystem reduction in reserve capacity, to the extent that a number of physiological systems are close to or past the threshold of symptomatic clinical failure'. As a consequence, the frail person is at increased risk of disability and death from minor external stresses. As age adds complexity to those with intellectual disability, common medical problems may have a greater effect on health and function in those with frailty than in younger people, and a comprehensive assessment is needed to manage frailty and maintain optimal function.

People with intellectual disability should attend their GP on a regular basis. Consideration should be given to the keeping of personal health records that remain the person's individual property – and so can be taken with them whenever there is a change of accommodation or service provider.

HEALTH SCREENING AND PREVENTION

Health screening and prevention activities are often neglected in those with intellectual disability of all ages and perhaps even more so in those who reach older age. There is evidence that continued screening programmes for mammography and cervical cancer are effective until later ages and most programmes recommend continued screening to age 75 years. Influenza vaccination is indicated for all persons aged 65 years and over, and in some countries pneumococcal vaccination is also indicated.

Lifestyle and health behaviours are important for the ageing person with intellectual disability. Smoking prevalence in people with mild intellectual disability may exceed that of the general population; however, people with intellectual disability are responsive to advice and education programmes on smoking cessation, with the majority quitting or reducing the amount they smoke.

Exercise can be undertaken by those with intellectual disability and is more important for all older people to maintain their cardiovascular health, functional status and general well-being. Thirty to 60 minutes of sustained low-level activity (such as walking) on at least three days per week will result in moderate health benefits such as reduced fatigue, weight loss, increased socialisation, improved control of Type 2 diabetes and less shortness of breath on exertion. No adverse effects of low to moderate activity have been observed in trials promoting physical activity for community-dwelling older people without disability. Advise regular, safe, physical activity as part of daily activities. Simple advice delivered in primary care is effective in increasing activity for older patients. Support persons and others involved in the care of older people with intellectual disability can facilitate activity programmes and these need to be included in general management plans. Recommend exercise that mimics the activities of daily living (such as repetitive sit to stand and walking). This type of exercise is more acceptable and beneficial for older people.

GENERAL MEDICAL ISSUES

Older people with intellectual disability experience the same health problems and associated ageing and lifestyle factors (exercise, diet, both active and passive smoking, drug and alcohol use) as any other older person; they require similar services from their doctors. Some conditions occur more frequently in older people with intellectual disability than in the general population. Common conditions are shown in Table 9.1.

TABLE 9.1 Medical and physical conditions common in older people with intellectual disability

Cardiorespiratory disorders	Gastrointestinal conditions:
Cerebrovascular disorders	gastro-oesophageal reflux disease
Hypertension	chronic constipation
Hyperlipidaemia	Incontinence
Diabetes	Urinary tract infections
Vision and hearing impairments	Cancer
Osteoporosis	Hypothyroidism
Arthritis	Parkinson's disease
Impaired mobility	Depression
Falls and fractures	Dementia

AGEING AND INTELLECTUAL DISABILITY SYNDROMES

Older people with intellectual disability experience health problems related to the aetiology of their disability and associated conditions. Some syndromes associated with intellectual disability are known to have specific health problems related to ageing. Adults with cerebral palsy experience physical changes attributed to ageing, including increased joint pain, decreased mobility and fatigue. Muscle mass loss and loss of elasticity associated with ageing are accentuated by the muscle shortening and increased muscle tone from upper motor neurone effects of cerebral palsy. Individuals with Down syndrome may also experience precocious ageing (early menopause, premature cataracts and presbycusis), and the incidence of Alzheimer's disease is higher in individuals with Down syndrome than the rest of the population (including those with intellectual disability).

MEDICATION REVIEW

All older people are at increased risk of adverse reactions due to complications from their medications. This issue causes up to 20% of hospitalisations for older people and has been the subject of national recommendations in at least one developed country. The UK National Service Framework recommends an annual review of medication for people aged 75 and over, with a six-monthly review for those taking four or more medicines. For further guidelines on medication review, *see* Chapter 10, 'Preventive Healthcare and Health Promotion' (p. 80).

SPECIFIC MEDICAL ISSUES
Cardiovascular and cerebrovascular disease

The incidence of cardiovascular – such as ischaemic heart disease and cardiac failure – and cerebrovascular disease in people with intellectual disability (excluding people who have Down syndrome) is thought to be similar to that of the general population. However, people with intellectual disability may not be the beneficiaries of public preventive health campaigns and are unlikely to present themselves for review and management of their vascular risk factors; therefore, it is important to actively identify, monitor and manage vascular risk factors in people with intellectual disability. The person with disability, and their families and other support persons, should be educated about healthy lifestyles and encouraged to implement dietary and exercise programmes. The long-term hypotensive effects of some psychotropic medications (e.g. chlorpromazine and thioridazine) also need to be considered.

There is some evidence that people with Down syndrome have lower rates of atherosclerosis and lower mean diastolic and systolic blood pressure than the general population. However, people with Down syndrome may have undiagnosed cardiac anomalies (including valvular and conduction defects) that may result in heart failure and other cardiac complications later in life.

Hypertension

Screening for and management of cardiovascular disease – and hypertension in particular – is more important for older people as they are at higher absolute risk of a cardiovascular event. Treatment of 10 older people with hypertension and diabetes, and 20 older people with hypertension, for five years will prevent one cardiovascular event. Hence, it is important to regularly screen older people with intellectual disability for hypertension.

Hyperlipidaemia

Consideration of lipid disorders is important for those with intellectual disability of all ages, as it is for the general population. If not previously considered or investigated, lipid levels should be measured in older adults.

Diabetes

Diagnosis and management of diabetes is often overlooked in people with intellectual disability. The prevalence of Type 2 diabetes increases with age. All people over 50 years of age are more likely to have diabetes (either diagnosed or undiagnosed). For those with intellectual disability, increased weight and low levels of exercise increase the risk of developing diabetes. Management is often complicated by difficulties in maintaining adequate levels of physical activity, adhering to dietary restrictions and implementing glucose monitoring (especially for people who are living independently or who are averse to pinpricks).

Vision and hearing impairment

Decline in vision and hearing is common in older people with intellectual disability. Sensory losses can result in social isolation, confusion and apparent loss of skill. Visual impairment may increase the risk of falls. Older adults with intellectual disability may be unable to report sensory losses and may be unaware of how such losses impact on their ability to function in their environment. In addition, support persons may attribute non-response to behavioural aspects (e.g. stubbornness) rather than to a sensory impairment. The following management strategies are recommended.

➤ Ensure regular hearing and vision assessments by service providers specialised in dealing with people with disability.
➤ Advise family members and other support persons on good communication practice; consult the local audiology services or a speech therapist.
➤ Ensure that support persons understand that older individuals require well-lit areas and glare-free environments in order to function safely and optimally.
➤ Referral to a speech therapist may be beneficial if communication is impaired by sensory loss or the individual is having difficulty in seeing or using their communication aid.

Skin and temperature homeostasis

Older people's skin becomes paler, wounds do not heal as quickly and skin becomes more vulnerable to sun damage. Adults with intellectual disability may not be aware of the importance of wearing sunscreen and that some medication (such as certain antipsychotics) may make them more vulnerable to sunburn.

A decrease in the number of sweat glands in the older individual means that heat dissipation is more difficult. In addition, age-associated breakdown in collagen and elastin fibres results in thinner, less pliable skin with less subcutaneous fat. This interferes with insulation and consequently older individuals are more susceptible to cold. Individuals with disability may not voice their discomfort and may not be able to rectify the situation themselves.

Older adults experience less thirst; therefore they have an increased risk of dehydration and heat stroke. The risk of dehydration in older adults with developmental disability may be increased as they may have difficulty drinking and may also avoid drinking in an effort to manage continence. The following management strategies are recommended.

➤ Provide health promotion on the importance of sunscreen and not staying out in the sun for long periods.
➤ Ensure that the individual and support persons understand the importance of adequate fluid intake during warm weather.
➤ Ensure that support persons are aware of the importance of monitoring an individual's body heat, and the need for the individual to avoid long periods unattended in either the sun or shade.

➤ Help support persons understand the importance of ensuring that the individual is warmly or coolly dressed (as appropriate) and that the need for more or less clothing can change quickly (e.g. moving from a sunny veranda into the house).

Gastrointestinal conditions

Constipation

The general population tends to lose bowel motility in the ageing process. Chronic constipation occurs in 50% to 85% of older people with intellectual disability, and is a particular problem for those who are non-ambulant. Severe constipation can result in both physical and behavioural problems. Monitoring bowel output regularly is important, as a change in bowel habit might be an indication of the development of bowel pathology. For more information *see* the constipation section in Chapter 8, 'Adult Healthcare' (p. 59).

Gastro-oesophageal reflux disease

For a discussion on gastro-oesophageal reflux disease in people with intellectual disability *see* Chapter 8, 'Adult Healthcare' (p. 58).

Urinary incontinence

Urinary incontinence is common in older people with intellectual disability, but is not part of the normal ageing process. It is usually caused by a treatable medical problem such as a urinary tract infection or other urological disorder, although it is commonly mistaken for a behavioural problem or attention seeking. A person with dementia may have problems locating or recognising the toilet; if they have dyspraxia, they may have difficulties at the toilet (e.g. with zips or buttons).

Communication difficulties, mobility and cognitive problems complicate management. Effective management of incontinence is important to minimise premature nursing home placement.

Arthritis

Arthritis is more prevalent in those with intellectual disability as muscle and joint disorders (particularly for those with cerebral palsy) increase with age in this population.

Management of arthritis in the older person with intellectual disability is complicated by the increased prevalence of comorbidities, more complex muscle and joint problems, and lesser amounts of regular physical activity. Effective common treatments for osteoarthritis of the knee include lower leg strengthening and aerobic exercise. Access to and compliance with this treatment may be more difficult for those with developmental disability.

Management of the pain of arthritis is complicated by the increased medication use as necessary for comorbidities. Caution should always be exercised when prescribing nonsteroidal anti-inflammatory agents (NSAIDs) in people also receiving angiotensin converting enzyme (ACE) inhibitors as renal toxicity is common, especially if furosemide is also being taken. NSAIDs can be used with caution and for short periods of time in older people, but the complication of gastrointestinal bleeding and renal impairment mean adverse reactions are common.

Osteoporosis, falls and fractures

Impairment in mobility is more common in older people with intellectual disability than in the general population. Their risk of falls is increased due to impaired mobility, coordination, balance, strength; epilepsy; the hypotensive and sedating effects of medications (especially psychotropic medications); and vision impairment. Older people with intellectual disability are also at greater risk of osteoporosis than older people in the general population because of:

➤ long-term mobility impairment and lack of weight-bearing exercise (due to physical disability or inadequate exercise programmes)
➤ inadequate dietary intake of calcium
➤ low vitamin D levels
➤ effects of long-term medications, such as antiepileptic or antipsychotic medications.

Those with hypogonadism or Down syndrome also have added risk of osteoporosis.

The combination of impaired mobility and osteoporosis increases the risk of fractures.

Community-dwelling older people with intellectual disability are at very high risk of falls and may benefit from proven preventive interventions. A programme of muscle strengthening and balance retraining, and advice on the use of assistive devices reduces the risk of falls by up to 50%. Local availability of falls clinics and falls-related exercise groups are variable. A 15-week course of Tai Chi Chuan exercises reduces falls by 50%; however, availability of classes may be limited. A review of all medical conditions, together with the treatment of cardiovascular disorders (particularly postural hypotension and cardiac arrhythmia), performing a medication review, and reducing psychotropic medications assists in preventing falls. Home safety assessment with modification of environmental hazards – usually by an occupational therapist – aids in preventing falls. Consider giving vitamin D and calcium to reduce the risk of vertebral fracture.

For older people in residential care who are at high risk of recurrent falls, referral to physiotherapy for gait and balance training and advice on the use of assistive devices aids mobility and assists in preventing falls. Medication review and reduction in medication use is more important in residential care. Give vitamin D and calcium to reduce the risk of hip fracture by 30%. Hip protective devices and garments are effective in reducing hip fracture.

The management of osteoporosis is discussed further on p. 62.

Hypothyroidism

Thyroid disease is important to rule out when evaluating a decline in overall functioning in a person with intellectual disability as they age. The symptoms of thyroid disease are more complex in older people and may present with general decline, weight gain, or non-specific symptoms. It is important to be alert to subtle changes in people with intellectual disability, especially as they age.

The management of hypothyroidism in older people is complicated by the higher prevalence of cardiovascular disorders. Introduction of thyroxine must be done with care. Starting at a low dose and titrating only every six weeks is recommended. Monitoring for arrhythmias (especially atrial fibrillation), congestive heart failure and other complications of thyroxine treatment is important.

Parkinson's disease

The management of Parkinson's disease is more complex as the patient ages because the adverse effects of medication (particularly postural hypotension, confusion and hallucinations) are both more common and cause greater morbidity in older age groups. Gradual dosage titration with vigilance given to adverse effects is more important for those with developmental disability, as symptoms may be expressed in unexpected ways. Extrapyramidal adverse effects of antipsychotic medication should not be confused with Parkinson's disease. The indication for, and dose of, antipsychotic medication should be reviewed before adding in anticholinergic or dopaminergic medications which can have significant effects on mental state.

PSYCHIATRIC ISSUES

The major psychiatric conditions to be considered in older people with intellectual disability are delirium, dementia, depression and chronic psychiatric disorders.

Delirium

Delirium has many causes including acute illness (commonly respiratory and urinary tract infections), metabolic disturbances, drug toxicity and withdrawal, and seizures. The hallmarks of delirium are acute or subacute onset, clouding of consciousness, impaired attention, fluctuating mental state, and disturbances in cognition, psychomotor activity, perception, emotional control and sleep-wake cycle. Delirium may be mistaken by support persons for a behavioural problem. It is important to identify and treat the underlying cause of the delirium. Medications should be reviewed for dosages, serum levels, potential for drug interactions and recent changes to the treatment regimen, particularly drugs with anticholinergic effects (e.g. propantheline for incontinence and benztropine for the treatment of extrapyramidal adverse effects of antipsychotic medication).

For those with intellectual disability, any change in functional status or fluctuation in usual self-care ability and behaviour should be taken seriously. As with all older people, symptoms of serious disease are masked by delirium, and easily treatable disorders can be missed. Accurate diagnosis of the cause of the delirium is essential and if this cannot be done in the community, referral for hospitalisation is recommended.

Dementia

By the age of 40 years, the typical neuropathological changes of Alzheimer's disease are present in those with Down syndrome – the average age of clinically diagnosable dementia is 50 years. However, rates of dementia in people with intellectual disability not due to Down syndrome are also higher than in the general population. The reason for this is not known; however, higher rates of vascular dementia are a possibility.

Diagnosis of dementia may be difficult as standard diagnostic tools (such as the Mini-Mental State Examination [MMSE]) are not validated for use in people with intellectual disability. Nonetheless, the MMSE may provide an individual benchmark for comparison over time in people with mild levels of intellectual disability. It is important to establish individual baseline functioning, and to demonstrate a clear deterioration (not due to another cause) over at least six months. Retrospective informant history is important but may not be reliable or available. It is important that those involved in the long-term care of people with developmental disability, especially people with Down syndrome, document a functional baseline. This could include standardised tests (such as the Vineland Adaptive Behaviour Scale) or detailed documentation of the ability to complete activities of daily living; this involves keeping samples of handwriting, artwork or drawings (e.g. 'draw-a-person' test), photographs of participation in activities, and even audio or videotaping. This will allow more reliable assessments of the nature and degree of any future decline.

If dementia is suspected, the work-up is similar to dementia work-ups in the general population. Functional decline may be due to many other common conditions; *see* Table 9.2. Hence, careful history taking, thorough medical assessment and sensory screening are essential.

TABLE 9.2 Differential diagnosis of functional decline in Down syndrome

Psychiatric and psychological disorder	Medical conditions
Depression	Hypothyroidism
Grief	Sleep apnoea
Adjustment disorders	Cardiac failure
Anxiety	Other
Delirium	
Psychosis	
Sensory impairments	**Medications**
Vision	Psychotropics
Hearing	Anticholinergics
	Polypharmacy

The clinical presentation of Alzheimer's disease in Down syndrome parallels the presentation in the general population, with:

➤ impairment of short-term memory and other cognitive functions
➤ decline in activities of daily living
➤ behavioural and psychological symptoms of dementia including changes in behaviour, personality and mood.

Alzheimer's disease is a predominantly temporoparietal disorder, hence identification of memory and language impairment, dyspraxia and visuospatial deficits are essential to making the diagnosis.

A history of repeated questioning (e.g. about who is on the next shift), forgetting names, or rummaging around looking for things, may all be indicative of memory impairment. Short-term memory impairment may be difficult to assess clinically in people who are non-verbal but may be assessed by hiding three objects in the room and testing the response to finding them.

The gradual decline in language (including losses in vocabulary, sentence complexity and spontaneity of communication) is a common presenting feature of Alzheimer's disease. A history of decline in daily living skills, and getting lost in familiar places, are additional clues to assist in a diagnosis of Alzheimer's disease. A distinction between trying to complete a task (and maybe being unable to) versus lack of motivation helps distinguish Alzheimer's disease from other causes of functional decline. A person who once neatly folded clothes but is now rolling them up may be showing signs of dyspraxia. Observing the person while they complete dressing tasks (e.g. taking off and putting on a jacket, undoing and doing buttons, tying up shoelaces) or manipulate a knife and fork can demonstrate dyspraxia. Impairment in visual and spatial skills may be demonstrated by a decline in the complexity and skill in artwork. Observations of drawing, writing and comparison with earlier artwork and writing can help identify decline in these areas.

Cholinesterase inhibitors

Cholinesterase inhibitors offer modest benefits to patients with mild to moderate dementia due to Alzheimer's disease. They are expensive, require supervision, improve alertness and function and maintain cognitive scores at or above the baseline for up to 12 months, but do not modify the underlying progression of pathology. Open-label trials have shown continued benefit for up to four years. Six-month studies suggest that between 5 and 15 patients need to be started on treatment in order to see a significant improvement in one patient. Two out of three treated patients have their apparent rate of cognitive decline slowed by cholinesterase inhibitor therapy. Patients should be treated for at least two months at the maximum tolerated dose of medication before a final assessment of response is made. There is no convincing evidence that any of the three available cholinesterase inhibitors is more efficacious than the other two; however, donepezil's once-daily dosing regimen and fewer adverse effects should make it the first choice medication for most patients. In the event of non-response, there is a lack of clear evidence to indicate that switching to another cholinesterase inhibitor will produce a response, though individual cases who respond to one drug but not to another have been described. There is a small body of evidence that cholinesterase inhibitors may be of benefit to people with Down syndrome and Alzheimer's disease.

The cholinesterase inhibitors are associated with prominent gastrointestinal adverse effects, particularly anorexia, nausea, vomiting and diarrhoea. Other possible adverse effects include insomnia, vivid dreams, asthma, bradyarrhythmias, cramps and dizziness. Care should be taken when introducing cholinesterase inhibitors in patients with asthma, chronic obstructive pulmonary disease, cardiac conduction abnormalities, peptic ulcer disease and when administering muscle relaxants to patients already taking a cholinesterase inhibitor. Galantamine is contraindicated in severe renal failure. Donepezil has a more favourable adverse effect profile, but the shorter half-lives of rivastigmine and galantamine may be advantageous in limiting the time course of adverse effects, if they occur. Drug interactions commonly occur.

Prior to commencing cholinesterase inhibitor treatment, it is important to do a thorough physical examination. People with Down syndrome who have Alzheimer's disease may not be able to report adverse effects of these medications. People with Down syndrome may have unsuspected cardiac problems including valvular and conduction defects. If there is a cardiac history or electrocardiogram (ECG) abnormalities, a cardiology review is recommended prior to commencing treatment. It is also important to monitor the patient, including weekly pulse and blood pressure measurement, during the first four weeks of treatment.

Depression, bereavement and grief

Depressive disorders are more common in older than younger people with intellectual disability, and this is particularly so in people with Down syndrome. In Down syndrome, depression may be related to the onset of Alzheimer's disease. Depression may result in loss of motivation, communication decline and functional decline. The distinction between depression and dementia may be difficult. If depressive symptoms are present, treatment with an antidepressant is recommended, followed by review of cognitive and daily function.

The assessment and management of depression are covered in Chapter 14, 'Assessment of Psychiatric Disorders', (p. 116) and Chapter 15, 'Management of Psychiatric Disorders', (p. 128). Antidepressants with significant anticholinergic effects (e.g. tricyclic antidepressants) should be avoided.

Old age is a time of loss and bereavement for people with intellectual disability just as for those without disability. Grief is often overlooked in people with intellectual disability and may result in significant levels of behavioural disturbance and psychopathology that may persist for a year or longer. Support, fostering understanding, expression of feelings, participation in the rites of passage and commemoration (e.g. photographs, visits and tending to the gravesite) are all-important in helping a person with intellectual disability to grieve. Continuing psychopathology and depression should be treated.

Chronic psychiatric disorders

Older people with intellectual disability may have chronic psychiatric disorders that are undiagnosed or misdiagnosed; psychotic disorders are overdiagnosed; mood disorders (such as bipolar disorder) are under-diagnosed. Psychotropic medications may not have been reviewed for many years, and the original indication may be long forgotten. It is, therefore, important to undertake a medication review, as described on p. 82.

Selective serotonin reuptake inhibitors (SSRIs) such as fluvoxamine, paroxetine and fluoxetine may inhibit metabolism of other psychotropics; this increases the risk of serious drug–drug interactions. High dosages of multiple antipsychotic medications indicate a lack of efficacy and are potentially dangerous, increasing the risk of sudden death. The diagnosis and treatment regimen should be reviewed. If the person has extrapyramidal adverse effects from antipsychotic medication, a review of the indication, reduction in dose or change to an atypical antipsychotic is preferable to using an anticholinergic medication (such as benztropine), as an anticholinergic may further impair cognition or even induce delirium. Antipsychotic medication should be withdrawn if there is no indication for its use.

Lighting

Although older individuals usually require more light to see adequately, they are susceptible to glare. Therefore, blinds and curtains that diffuse light may be helpful. Shiny polishes and paints should be avoided, especially in kitchens and bathrooms.

Noise

Background noise may be a problem, particularly in institutions or shared houses. Conversations in a noisy environment (e.g. with music playing or noisy appliances) should be avoided if the individual has any hearing impairment.

Manual dexterity

Any decrease in manual dexterity may make opening bottles, jars and doors more difficult. This applies to the ageing support person just as much as to the individual with intellectual disability. Opening of childproof medication or blister packs may be problematic – in such cases the doctor can request that medication be dispensed into a Dosette or similar container.

Modifications to the environment

Environmental modification and simple safety measures (e.g. bathroom doors that open outwards, the addition of ramps and rails, equipment such as a wheelchair or scooter) may make the difference between a person remaining at home and being moved into institutional care. There is an obligation by the community to support the person with intellectual disability and their ageing support persons in obtaining environmental modification and equipment that will enable them to have an optimal quality of life.

PLACEMENT IN AGED CARE FACILITIES

For some older people with intellectual disability who are infirm or have advanced dementia, placement in a nursing home is appropriate. However, older people with intellectual disability are a survivor population who are relatively healthy and have high levels of adaptive functioning. As a group, they are less likely to have gone to school or to have worked, have less community and family contact, and have high rates of institutional and nursing home care. Some older people have never had contact with disability services as all their care has been provided by the family. Future planning for older people with developmental disability living with ageing parents is important but difficult due to limited accommodation options. Parents are often not able to accept residential care for their child. It is not uncommon for older people to be placed in an aged care facility when family caregivers are no longer able to provide care. Placement in an aged care facility may be precipitous, due to the sudden decline in health or the death of the family caregiver, and the person with the developmental disability may have no age-related physical or mental decline. Grief and being in an environment that does not cater to the person's social, emotional and activity needs may result in behaviours that staff and others find 'challenging'. It is important to resist the pressure to use psychotropic medications for social problems.

To illustrate with an example: a 67-year-old man with mild intellectual disability and no health problems was placed in a nursing home when his mother could no longer care for him; he became emotionally attached to an ill elderly lady with dementia and his devotion to her was not in her best interests. A day placement was arranged and the problem resolved.

Placement in hostel settings may be problematic. While the person may be independent in self-care they may not be able to cope with the relatively unstructured environment of the hostel. This may lead to challenging behaviours and placement breakdown. If the hostel is not able to provide more structured care, placement in a community residential unit should be sought.

FURTHER READING

- Cooper SA. Epidemiology of psychiatric disorders in elderly compared with younger adults with learning disabilities. *Br J Psychiatry.* 1997; **170**: 375–80.
- Cooper SA. Clinical study of the effects of age on the physical health of adults with mental retardation. *Am J Ment Retard.* 1998; **102**(6): 582–9.
- Hollins S, Attard MT, von Fraunhofer N, *et al.* Mortality in people with learning disability: risks, causes, and death certification findings in London. *Dev Med Child Neurol.* 1998; **40**(1): 50–6.
- Patja K, Iivanainen M, Vesala H, Oksanen H, Ruoppila I. Life expectancy of people with intellectual disability: a 35-year follow-up study. *J Intellect Disabil Res.* 2000; **44**(5): 591–9.

CHAPTER 10

Preventive healthcare and health promotion

In a population that does not communicate well (and contains people who do not complain), preventive healthcare and general screening for disease and relevant risk factors is more important than in people without disability (e.g. people with intellectual disability will rarely request vaccination or the measurement of cholesterol levels, and support persons may be reluctant to suggest tests). Although people with intellectual disability drink alcohol and smoke less frequently than other people, the minority who do smoke or drink benefit from health education. General health screening (of cholesterol and glucose levels) and lifestyle advice should be more frequent than in the non-disabled population.

YEARLY PHYSICAL

There is clear irrefutable evidence that an annual formal physical examination by a GP will detect previously undetected disease in at least 9% patients seen, and will increase the rates of screening and immunisation.

HEALTH SCREENING

General screening tests should be performed according to the same indications and contraindications as the general population. Table 10.1 lists the recommended tests for adults, and their frequencies.

Certain tests may be traumatic for people with intellectual disability; an assessment of the relative risks and benefits should be made in each case.

Cervical cytology and mammography are poorly accessed by people with disability. Cervical cytology (Pap smears) is not required for women who have never been sexually active. However, breast examination and mammography is indicated at the appropriate time for all women with intellectual disability. *See also* Chapter 21, 'Women's Health' (p. 171).

Regular inspection of genitalia should be part of the physical examination of males.

Special screening tests are indicated, as with the general population, where there is a family history of heritable diseases such as colon cancer, familial hypercholesterolaemia and glaucoma. Whenever possible, obtain details of family history from relatives (as paid support persons may be unaware of them).

TABLE 10.1 Adult healthcare checklist and recommended screening frequency

Health issues	Screening frequency
Blood pressure check	Yearly
Dental check	Six-monthly
Hearing assessment	Every three to five years by an audiologist
Vision assessment	Every three to five years by an optometrist/ ophthalmologist
Medication review	Regularly review indications and adverse effects
Thyroid function test	Down syndrome – yearly
Hyperlipidaemia	Non-Down syndrome – yearly or less frequently (depending on aetiological diagnosis)
Diabetes	Regularly review
	Regularly review
Lifestyle	
Alcohol intake review	Yearly
Tobacco intake review	Yearly*
Diet review	Yearly
Weight review	Yearly
Exercise review	Yearly
Sleep pattern review	Yearly
Examination for skin tumours	Yearly
Women's health	
Breast examination	GP to regularly review (frequency not clearly established)
Mammography	Every two years after the age of 50
Pap smear	If patient has ever been sexually active – every two years between the ages of 18 and 70
Men's health	
Screen for cryptoorchidism	On first presentation
Inspect genitalia	Yearly
Immunisation	
Hepatitis A	If indicated
Hepatitis B	If indicated
Influenza	If indicated – yearly
Pneumococcal	If indicated
Diphtheria/tetanus	Primary course and 10-yearly
Other	
Epilepsy	Continual awareness of risk. If on antiepileptics consider the need for vitamin D supplementation
Incontinence	Diagnose and treat cause of changes
Mobility	Continual monitoring; address changes
Problem behaviour	If indicated – consider physical/psychological/social issues
Psychiatric disorder	Continual awareness of risk
Sexual health	If indicated, offer advice on contraception and safe sex
Episode of low-trauma fracture	Measure bone mineral density

* Most reports show a low incidence of smoking but more recent reports indicate rates the same as the rest of the population in those with mild and moderate intellectual disability.

NUTRITION

There is a greater prevalence of obesity (up to 27%) in people with intellectual disability compared to the general population; poor diet and lack of exercise are significant contributors and obesity often remains unmanaged. Being underweight is also common and often requires intervention. Other nutritional problems include osteomalacia, vitamin D and B_{12} deficiency and poor dietary calcium intake. For more information *see* Chapter 8, 'Adult Healthcare' (p. 62) and Chapter 17, 'Nutritional Disorders' (p. 146).

EXERCISE

Studies confirm the comparative inactivity of people with intellectual disability, and the degree of inactivity ranges greatly. The non-ambulant person (e.g. one with spastic quadriplegia who is confined to bed or a wheelchair) requires referral to allied health professionals; ambulant people (who may, despite being physically able to exercise, lack the opportunities or motivation to exercise) benefit from formal exercise programmes.

IMMUNISATION

All people with intellectual disability should be vaccinated according to the standard schedule. Researchers have shown that people with intellectual disability are less likely to be vaccinated against tetanus, diphtheria, poliomyelitis and influenza.

Documentation of previous vaccination history may not be obtainable. Older people and those who have had several residential placements often do not have complete (or any) health records. Where few records exist catch-up vaccination is important. Detailed advice about catch-up vaccination is contained in *Immunisation Against Infectious Disease – 'The Green Book'* (Department of Health, UK).

Vaccination against influenza and pneumococcal disease is especially important because of the high mortality of this population from respiratory disease. Annual influenza vaccination is recommended for all people over 65 years of age, children and adults with chronic illnesses requiring regular medical follow-up, and residents of nursing homes and other long-term care facilities.

Hepatitis A and B vaccination is recommended for people with intellectual disability and their support persons, especially if they live in group settings. Hepatitis B vaccination is also recommended for household contacts of acute and chronic hepatitis B carriers.

Pneumococcal vaccination is indicated for all individuals over 65 years of age, indigenous people over 50 years, the immunocompromised, and immunocompetent people with chronic disease such as diabetes, cardiac, pulmonary or renal disease.

MEDICATION REVIEW

People with intellectual disability are often on multiple medications, especially psychotropics and antiepileptics. Medication regimens may not have changed for many years. Some medications may no longer be indicated, and modern, safer and better tolerated alternatives may be available. Other medications may be maintained at unnecessarily high dosages. Often, because of difficulty in obtaining a past history, it may not be possible to determine the original reason for the prescribing of certain medications. If there is no clear current indication for a medication, it should be cautiously withdrawn.

As people with intellectual disability age, they are likely to develop medical problems requiring additional medications. This occurs at a time when the capacity to metabolise and excrete drugs may be declining. There is much potential for drug–drug interactions and for the occurrence of adverse effects of increased serum levels of medications. Hence the indication for, and the dose of, medications should be regularly reviewed, at intervals of three to 12 months, *see* Box 10.1.

BOX 10.1 Points for consideration when undertaking a medication review

What is the diagnosis and indication for treatment?
Is the medication treating the diagnosis – or only modifying symptoms of the disorder?
Dosage – consider potentially dangerous doses
Efficacy
Adverse effects
Route (e.g. depot in an orally compliant patient)
Possible alternative medications
Potentially dangerous doses or combinations

ABUSE

People with intellectual disability are particularly vulnerable to sexual abuse (both men and women may be victims), psychological abuse and physical abuse; all of which may remain unrecognised and be left untreated. Abuse may occur in the person's school, work or home environment, and may contribute to the development of a psychiatric disorder or behavioural problem. For more information on dealing with victims of sexual abuse, *see* Chapter 20, 'Sexuality' (p. 166).

FURTHER READING

- Kerr MP. Primary health care for people with an intellectual disability. *J Intellect Disabil Res.* 1997; **41**(5): 363–4.
- Lennox N, Rey-Conde T, Bain C, *et al*. The evidence for better health from health assessments: a large clustered randomised controlled trial. *J Intellect Disabil Res.* 2004; **48**: 343.

CHAPTER 11

Annual health checks

Annual checks for adults with intellectual disability have long been known to be effective in preventing illness and promoting an improved quality of life. Of 181 Welsh adults with intellectual disabilities receiving structured health checks, new clinical needs were identified in 51%, of whom 25% had two new needs and 12% more than two needs identified; 9% (16 patients) of the total had serious new morbidity.

In a one-year period 50 participants offered a health screen intervention in Glasgow were individually matched with 50 who were offered standard general practice care only. In the intervention group, 4.80 new clinical needs were identified, compared with 2.26 in the group receiving standard treatment only. The level of met new health needs was also greater, 3.56 vs. 2.26. The 10 conditions showing the greatest difference in frequency of needs detection between the intervention and standard group were mental ill health, impacted wax, urine infection/prostatism, cataracts/visual impairment, gastro-oesophageal reflux disorder, arthritis, eczema, hearing impairment, hypertension and drug side-effects.

The following system (*see* Table 11.1) of undertaking the check has been developed in view of two basic criteria:
1 It should be administered by the primary care team (with support from specialist learning disability services, where available). Thus the two basic clinicians always involved would be practice nurse and GP.
2 It should be computer system compatible.

This annual clinical needs assessment for patients with intellectual disabilities (ACNAPID) has been structured to be comprehensive yet adaptable to the actual needs of people with learning disabilities and their carers. Initially, the patient will be comprehensively assessed, with completion of all sections. Section A will only need completion at initial check. Section B will always be completed annually; usually this will be best administered by the practice nurse. There could be needs identified in some or each subsection of Section C. For example, it would be advisable to check carefully sections about epilepsy, ambulation and reflux in patients with cerebral palsy (*see* sections A and C). On the other hand, where an initial check fails to identify any activity in section C and the patient does not require medication review, the practice nurse with access to a GP may be able to administer subsequent checks.

The checks are designed to be administered without any particular specialist knowledge of intellectual disability. In section C (paper version), the questions, usually at the beginning of sections, are 'excluding type' questions, and if negative, should lead the clinician directly to the next subsection.

DOCUMENTATION

There will be three phases to this:
1 An input invitation and patient agenda document.
2 The clinical assessment.
3 An output/implementation document.

1 Invitation and patient's agenda

This separate document would be sent to the patient's residence for completion and should accompany the patient when they (and carers) attend for the assessment.

2 The clinical assessment

BOX 11.1 Clinical assessment

> **Section A: Important background information**
> Demographic details
> Diagnosis of condition
> Communication
> Consent
>
> **Section B: General health check**
> Well person/lifestyle check
> Screening, contraception
> Immunisations
>
> **Section C: Specific health needs assessment**
> Nervous System, etc
> Sight
> Hearing
> Epilepsy
> Mental Illness
> Behavioural
> Musculoskeletal
> Alimentary System
> Genitourinary System
> Miscellaneous
> Metabolic
> Medications
> Blood Tests

3 Implementation document

This should be agreed by those present and should set out how identified interventions will be actioned, and who is responsible for implementation. It may be a written document, and could be computer-generated.

ANNUAL CLINICAL NEEDS ASSESSMENT FOR PATIENTS WITH INTELLECTUAL DISABILITIES

The paper version uses a Y/N format; usually the right-hand letter, N or Y, indicates a problem or area where intervention may be needed. *See* Table 11.1.

FURTHER READING

- Baxter H, Lowe K, Houston H, *et al*. Previously unidentified morbidity in patients with intellectual disability. *Br J Gen Pract*. 2006; **56**: 93–8.
- Cooper SA, Morrison J, Melville C, *et al*. Improving the health of people with intellectual disabilities: outcomes of a health screening programme after 1 year. *J Intellect Disabil Res*. 2006; **50**: 667–77.
- Felce D, Baxter H, Lowe K, *et al*. The impact of repeated health checks for adults with intellectual disabilities. *J Appl Res Intellect Disabil*. 2008; **10**(1111/j): 1468–3148.
- Felce D, Baxter H, Lowe K, *et al*. The impact of checking the health of adults with intellectual disabilities on primary care consultation rates, health promotion and contact with specialists. *J Appl Res Intellect Disabil*. 2008; **10**(1111/j): 1468–3148.
- Hoghton MA and RCGP Learning Disabilities Group. Step by step guide for GP practices: annual health checks for people with a learning disability. RCGP; 2010.
- Lennox N, Bain C, Rey-Conde T, *et al*. Effects of a comprehensive health assessment programme for Australian adults with intellectual disability: a cluster randomized trial. *Int J Epidemiol*. 2007; **30**: 139–46.

TABLE 11.1 Annual clinical needs assessment for patients with intellectual disabilities

MAIN SECTIONS: Section A	PAPER VERSION	READ CODE VERSION LD Health Assessment 9HB3.00	ACTION
		* * *	* *
UNDERLYING CONDITION AND LEVEL OF ID	Record Diagnosis and level of disability. Record underlying disability, e.g. Down syndrome, fragile X syndrome, cerebral palsy, autistic spectrum disorder, neural tube disorder, or rarer identified conditions. If underlying condition unknown, record if patient refused investigation or whether recent investigation has failed to identify cause.	Record diagnosis and level of disability in *Diagnosis window. Read Codes currently available for Intellectual Disability include the E3 and Eu7. (Eu7 may be stratified into mild Eu70, moderate Eu71 severe Eu72 and profound Eu73. Both codes have the underlying concept of intellectual disability, though both are currently described by the obsolete 'mental retardation' epithet. At present it is unnecessary for GP register purposes, to record level of ID.) If ID underlying diagnosis established, 1a] should be skipped at future annual checks.*	
COMMUNICATION CONSENT	No speech problems? If communication difficulties, record degree and preferred methods of communication; initial check only. Comprehension level? Method of/capacity to consent? Usually agree with proposition? How express disapproval?	Y N No speech problems Speech problems Problems with communication, incl. speech Communication skills Refer to speech and language Obtaining consent Verbal consent for examination Method of consent; verbal/non-verbal/best interests	1B91 1B9 ZV401 13o. 8H7G 9Nd 9Nd0
SUMMARY			

(continued)

GENERAL
Section B — HEALTH CHECK

	HEALTH CHECK		
WELL PERSON	BP....../.........bpm	BP, Pulse rhythm	243
	Pulse............bpm	Weight/weight change from baseline	
LIFESTYLE	Weight.........kg		
MANAGEMENT	wt change from baseline	Height, BMI	22K
PLAN	Height......m	waist circum	22N0
	BMI......	Smoking	1371
	Smoking.............cig/d	Alcohol consumption	136..00
	Alcohol..........u/wk	Exercise grading	138..00
	Exercise.........	Diet enquiry and advice	8CA4.
	Diet.........	Use standard well person check grid	
	Appropriate advice and follow up should be arranged, e.g. for obesity. Also patient/carer concerns/agenda should be discussed at this point.	*Patient/carer concerns/agenda should be discussed at this point, and actions recorded for health action plan (HAP)*	
		No code for patient concerns/agenda	
SCREENING	Check appropriate screening done after necessary counselling/ preparation.	Check appropriate screening done after necessary counselling/preparation/consent. Screening	68
	Cervical cytology	N Cervical cytology	685
	Mammogram	N Mammogram	6862
	Testicular check; patient doing self-examination or carer inspection?	Y Y Y N Testicular check; patient doing self-examination or carer inspection?	679B.
IMMUNISATIONS	Check immunisations up to date? If not, arrange implementation. Flu? Hep B, Hep A, Pheu, Other?	Y N *View immunisation summary screen and offer to implement those due, or incomplete.*	2J6
SUMMARY OF NEEDS; ACTIONS			

SPECIFIC Section C — HEALTH NEEDS ASSESSMENT

SENSORY VISION

Vision normal? R L	Y N	Normal vision	6668A
Date of last optician review?.............		Seen by optician	9N2U
Eye discomfort?	Y	Eye discomfort? Visual symptoms	1B7A.00
Cataract present? RE/LE	Y	O/e cataract	22E5
Eligible blind/part-sighted registered?	Y	Visual aid?	8D3
	N	Blind/part-sighted register?	
Consider referring to eye surgeon for cataract, registration or other problems.			

HEARING

Hearing normal?	Y N	Hearing normal	1C11
Examination of ears normal?	Y N	Ears normal	2D13.
Hearing problems? R L	N Y	Hearing difficulty	1C12
Impacted wax? R L	N Y	Wax	2D82./F504
Arrange syringing. Prescribe oil.			
Change/reduction in hearing?	N Y	H/O poor hearing?	1493
Consider referral to consultant		Refer other doctor.	8H6
ENT/Hearing Aid Fitter/SALT assessment.		Hearing aid worn	2DG
		*	

EPILEPSY

Epilepsy or h/o Epilepsy?	N Y	H/o Epilepsy	1473.
Active epilepsy?	N Y	Epilepsy	F25.
Under consultant supervision?	Y N	Specialist supervision?	
Record details of current types of seizures, frequencies, investigations, actions, medication?*		Seizures	667.
		Seizure free >1year	667F.
		Fit frequency	6675.
Written seizure protocol?	N Y	Written protocol?	

(continued)

SPECIFIC Section C — **HEALTH NEEDS ASSESSMENT**

SPECIFIC Section C	HEALTH NEEDS ASSESSMENT	Y/N		Code
MENTAL ILLNESS	No evidence of mental illness?	Y	No evidence of mental illness	1I4.
	Known mental health problems?	N Y	History of psychiatric disorder?	146.
	Current consultant supervision?	Y N	Under specialist supervision?	
	On mental health register/CPA	N Y	Mental Health review?	6A6./1P52
			On severe mental illness register	9H8./146B.
	Depression present?	Y N	Depression	
	Dementia present?	N Y	Dementia?	
	Other mental illness present?	N	Other mental illness present?	
BEHAVIOUR, ETC	Behaviour disturbance/change?	N Y	Behaviours and observations related to behaviour	
	Specify/record nature...............		1P....	
	Normal sleep pattern?		Behaviour assessment	3AB.
		Y N	Behaviour change?	3AB3.
	Hours asleep?.........		Poor sleep pattern	1B1Q.
MUSCULO-SKELETAL	**Ambulation problems?**	N Y	Fully mobile?	13C1.00
	Describe problems briefly..........		Fair/poor/housebound	13C1.00 A/E/G
	Posture normal?	Y N	O/e posture normal	2981.
	Ask walking distance................ metres		Mobility assessment	398..
			Mobility screen	680..
	Decrease since previous year?	N Y	Mobility equipment requested	8M42
	Aids used?	Y Y	Dependent on wheelchair	ZV462
	Wheelchair; crutches; splints; boots? Consider referral to physiotherapist, orthopaedic surgeon chiropodist, or appliances fitter for review/advice.		Refer to physio	8H77.
			Chiropody care needed?	8D46
			Refer chiropodist	2L83./8H7R.
	Feet: inspect as indicated.		O/E foot.................	2G5..
	Consider referrals; treat arthritis, musculoskeletal pain, infections.		C/o foot symptom	1D28.

SPECIFIC
Section C

HEALTH NEEDS ASSESSMENT

Category	Question			Description	Code
ALIMENTARY SYSTEM	Regular dental review arranged?	Y	N	Dental examination?	3165.
	Date of last review?..........			Date of last review? o/e teeth and	2541.
	Dental/oral problem identified?	N	Y	Problem identified? Refer or treat as above	
	Dysphagia present?	N	Y	Dysphagia symptoms	194..
	Lung aspiration possible?	N	Y	Lung aspiration suspected?	
	Reflux/dyspepsia suspected?	N	Y	Reflux oesophagitis	J1011
	H. pylori test indicated?	N	Y	*H. pylori* serology positive	4DJ6.
	H. pylori eradication treatment given?	N	Y	*H. pylori* eradication treatment	8BAC.
	Diarrhoea/constipation?	N	Y	Constipation	J52Q.
	Incontinence?	N	Y	Incontinent	3932
	If Y for any consider diet advice, investigation, refer dietician/ medication.			Treatment indicated	8BQ..
				Refer dietician	8H76..
				Investigation indicated	8BR..
UROGENITAL Urinary	Urinalysis including sugar, protein, blood, leucocytes normal?	Y	N	Urinalysis	461..12
				Fully continent	3940
	Continence problem?	N		Incontinent	3942.
	Consider referral to continence adviser.			Occasional incontinence	3941.
	Could continence/enuresis be improved?			Refer to continence adviser	8H7W
	If yes; treat/refer appropriately.				
GYNAECOLOGICAL	**Gynaecological symptoms?**	N	Y	GU symptoms?	1A...
	Amenorrhoea? FSH necessary	N	Y	Amenorrhoea	1571.
	Menorrhagia? Hb?/Fe therapy?	N	Y	Menorrhagia	1573
	Other symptoms?			Other gynaecological symptoms	157..
	(dysmen, discharge, PMB, IMB).	N	Y	PMT	K584.
	Investigate/treat as required;				
	PMT treatment, HRT, indicated?	N	Y	HRT	

(continued)

SPECIFIC Section C	HEALTH NEEDS ASSESSMENT			
METABOLIC, MISC OTHER CONDITIONS NOT MENTIONED ELSEWHERE	Lethargy/ tiredness present? Consider TFT/Hb for Down syndrome, etc, also if lethargy, unexplained weight gain?	N	Y	Lethargy TFT	168.. 442..13
	Osteoporosis suspected?	N	Y	At risk of osteoporosis	1409.
	History of fracture? FH? Height loss? Investigate and treat by local protocols, including Dexa Scan.	N	Y	DXA scan heel	8HQC..
	Osteoporosis present	N	Y	Osteoporosis	N330.00
	Skin problems?	N	Y	Dermatology	2F.1.
MEDICATIONS	On repeat medication? N/Y Refer to acute and repeat drug screens or repeat prescription counterfoils.	N	Y	On Repeat medication? Refer to acute and repeat drug screens Epilepsy medication review	8B1F.
	AEDs and hormones: side-effects?		Y	Any evidence of side-effects?	
	Could dosage be adjusted or withdrawn?	N	Y	Could any drug dosage be adjusted or withdrawn? Analgesics /NSAIDs needed?	
	Any acute treatments indicated? Any analgesics of NSAIDs indicated?	N	Y	Discussion about treatment (any)	8CP..
BLOOD TESTS	Consider TFT, Hb, FSH, Lithium, Cholesterol Anticonvulsant levels			Consider TFT, Hb, Cholesterol, anticonvulsant levels or Lithium,	
COMMENTS				LD Action plan offered	9HB0.00

CHAPTER 12

Challenging behaviour

People with intellectual disability have a high prevalence of challenging behaviours that are major contributors to social isolation, skill impairment and distress. Challenging behaviours limit accommodation and employment opportunities and are very costly in terms of support people's stress, injury and higher staff ratios, thereby limiting the ability of people with developmental disability to live full and happy lives.

Challenging behaviours are, according to Emerson (1995) 'behaviours of such intensity, frequency or duration that the physical safety of the person or others is placed in serious jeopardy or behaviour which is likely to seriously limit or deny access to the use of ordinary community facilities'.

Challenging behaviours include:
➤ aggression
➤ property destruction
➤ self-injurious behaviour
➤ socially inappropriate behaviour
➤ withdrawn behaviour
➤ repetitive behaviour
➤ non-compliant behaviour.

In the past there was a tendency to ascribe these behaviours to the person's underlying intellectual and developmental disability; however, while the person's disability may be a contributing factor, the clinician should always consider precipitating social, medical or psychiatric factors. Where the person presents with loss of skills then an underlying organic cause needs to be excluded.

Examples of commonly observed challenging behaviours are:
➤ A person with severe intellectual disability hitting themselves about the face and head, causing bruising and open wounds.
➤ A person with mild intellectual disability becoming uncooperative and abusive with support persons.
➤ A person with autism and moderate intellectual disability refusing to go to a public place, and if taken becoming aggressive and running away from support people.

➤ A person with mild intellectual disability becoming withdrawn and lethargic, and complaining of stomach pain and nausea.

MANAGEMENT

As challenging behaviour often has a number of contributing factors, effective management involves a team approach and the clinician needs to use systematic methodology. Consider referral options early in the management – it is best to act early as there may be substantial waiting lists and it may take a while to find the best option. The checklist for assessment (Table 12.1) is a useful assessment guide to follow:

TABLE 12.1 Checklist for assessment

Step by step

1 Assess the safety of your patient and everybody who lives and works with them.

2 Describe the challenging behaviour including frequency, duration, setting and severity.

3 Address the support person's needs and limitations.

4 Perform a medical and psychiatric assessment and continue information gathering.

5 Integrate other resources and assessments.

6 Review and plan intervention.

7 Manage and refer.

8 Monitor and review.

1 Safety

Safety is the first priority. People with intellectual disability have a high risk of injury and abuse, and those with challenging behaviour are at greatest risk. It may take days or weeks to solve the puzzle of the challenging behaviour; in the meantime, everybody needs to be and feel safe.

Temporary containment, restraint and sedation

Constraints and/or sedation may be necessary for a short time; it is important that these are temporary. Many times so-called 'temporary measures' designed to contain a difficult situation turn into a way of life for people with intellectual disability. An example is the ongoing prescription of sedating medication, often an antipsychotic drug. Any form of restraint may have legal implications, and should never be envisaged as a permanent solution.

Protection

A person with intellectual disability may also need protection from others; when displaying challenging behaviour they are at increased risk of injury by stressed support persons, or bewildered and anxious house and work mates.

Emergency plan

Having a plan in place for what to do and who to call when a situation becomes unsafe promotes a feeling of safety. Help support persons to develop an emergency plan and reach agreement with their colleagues about its content.

2 Describing behaviour

Many terms used to describe the state of a disturbed person provide limited information about the actual behaviour (e.g. agitated, inappropriate, deviant, restless). A comprehensive assessment begins with the clearest description of the behaviour and its frequency, setting, duration and severity. For example:

➤ Behavioural overview: aggressive – hitting people with fists.
➤ Frequency: on three days out of the last five – two episodes a day.
➤ Setting: at the day centre.
➤ Duration: for 10 minutes.
➤ Severity: 5 on a 5-point scale – others have been injured (e.g. bruised).

Many terms for symptoms used in medical assessments may be difficult to explain to, or have described by, a person with developmental disability. The concept of behavioural equivalents is useful in this context; it refers to observable behaviour, which (if present) may suggest the presence of the symptom of interest (*see* Table 12.2). Support persons can observe and document the frequency, duration, setting and severity of relevant behaviours.

TABLE 12.2 Behavioural equivalents examples

Symptom of interest	Behavioural equivalents
Worry	Repeated questioning
Restlessness	Pacing up and down
Muscle tension	Clenched fists
Dry mouth	Frequent drinks
Nausea	Food refusal

Another way to describe behaviour is to use a checklist. The Developmental Behaviour Checklist, which is available in versions for children and adults with intellectual disability, is a well-researched Australian instrument that support persons can easily complete. The checklist contains a comprehensive list of challenging behaviours and is completed at intervals by support persons who know the person with developmental disability well; it can be used to document changes in behaviour over time or in response to specific interventions.

3 Limitations and needs of carers

Carers often accompany a person with significant intellectual impairment to an appointment with a health professional. They may be a family member, a friend or an employee of an organisation and can be an invaluable source of information and assistance. Support persons themselves might have needs that require assistance from the GP. If the carer does not know the person with intellectual disability well, the support person may be of little or no assistance; and occasionally they may be a contributor to the presenting concern.

Misconceptions of support persons

A carer may be poorly informed ('I'm a temporary staff member just on today'), unfamiliar with the current problem ('I just returned from leave today'), or there may be disagreements between carers about the problem ('It never happens when I'm there'). It is useful to cross check information with a range of support people and let agencies know when work practices are interfering with an assessment.

Attitudes to sexual expression

People with intellectual disability may have little (if any) personal space or privacy, and support persons may have a low tolerance for any form of sexual behaviour. Sexual behaviour that injures no one is everybody's right. The support person's concern in this area may not be legitimate but rather reflecting their own discomfort. For more information *see* Chapter 20, 'Sexuality' (p. 163).

Acceptance of developmentally normal behaviour

Carers may not appreciate the limitations of low intellectual functioning and may persist in expecting different behaviour or changes in behaviour that are not realistic. For example, a few people with intellectual disability never achieve complete toilet training and no amount of 'behavioural modification' or other treatment changes the situation.

Stressed carers

Paid and unpaid carers experience times of stress in their caring role, when a usual or 'normal' situation of somebody's behaviour becomes too difficult for them to cope with. Carers also have their own health and lifestyle issues.

Solutions to consider

There are several strategies that may help support persons:
➤ Coordinate support person management – consistency in approaching the situation helps everybody.
➤ Organise respite care for people with developmental disability and their support persons.
➤ Address health needs and lifestyle issues of support persons.
➤ Educate support persons
  – so that expectations are realistic
  – to become familiar with and comply with legislation
  – to develop stress management strategies.

4 Medical and psychiatric assessment, and continued information gathering

Medical assessment

The cognitive and communication problems associated with intellectual disability may result in a difference in the way that medical problems present in people with intellectual disability. Research has established the importance of a thorough medical assessment in people with intellectual disability who present with challenging behaviour. The medical assessment is important to identify not only potential causes and factors that perpetuate challenging behaviour but also associated medical problems and risks that may result from the behaviour.

ASSESSMENT OF BEHAVIOURAL HISTORY

Before making a medical and psychiatric assessment, the clinician should carefully consider and document the history of the challenging behaviour. The assessment may provide a basis for making a diagnosis or directing further investigation. Table 12.3 lists questions that will help obtain a detailed history of the behaviour.

TABLE 12.3 Questions to guide the establishment of a challenging behaviour history

General questions	Further prompts
When is the behaviour most likely to occur?	What is the relationship to meal times? Is it worse at night?
What happens immediately prior to the behaviour?	Where is the person? What are they doing? What are others doing?
Does any activity or event make the behaviour more likely?	Is the behaviour more likely with exercise? Does it follow eating certain foods?
What is the long-term history of the behaviour?	Does it follow certain medical events or has it occurred in association with a particular medical problem? Has the behaviour always been present but not at the current severity?
Is there a medical cause for the behaviour?	What is the underlying cause for the developmental disability? What is the past medical history? Are there associated medical disorders that could explain the behaviours?

FOCUS ON AREAS OF CONCERN

Follow the general behavioural history with a careful systems review that includes more focused attention on areas of concern identified through the presenting history, past medical history and the underlying cause for the developmental disability. Particular attention should be given to symptoms of epilepsy and, if there is a history of seizures, determine the seizure frequency and their effect on behaviour. Sometimes a comprehensive physical examination is difficult to achieve, and whether to progress with it warrants careful consideration of the potential risks and benefits before more invasive investigations are carried out.

In considering potential medical causes for challenging behaviour a systematic approach is often advisable. The diagnostic model proposed by Murtagh can be applied to all patients; it is also a useful guide to the assessment and diagnosis of patients with challenging behaviour:

1 **The probability diagnosis**: utilises knowledge of common conditions that occur at specific ages (e.g. an impacted wisdom tooth in a 20-year-old autistic male presenting with head banging; dysmenorrhoea in a 35-year-old woman with intellectual disability and aggressive outbursts prior to and during her periods; dementia in a non-compliant and agitated 55-year-old man with Down syndrome).

2 **Serious conditions that should not be missed** should then be considered, including neoplasia (particularly malignancy), serious infections, cardiovascular and cerebrovascular disease. Cardiovascular disease may present late and should be considered in an older patient who is struggling with physical work or exercise (e.g. an obese 45-year-old man with a strong family history of cardiovascular disease who starts refusing to go on walks during his day programme).

3 **Problems that are commonly missed**: the importance of considering Murtagh's 'pitfalls' (i.e. problems that are commonly missed) applies equally well to people with intellectual disability. These include drug reactions, domestic abuse, seizure disorders, faecal impaction, urinary tract infection, migraines, oesophagitis and menopausal symptoms. While all of these problems are relatively common in people with intellectual disability, they are more difficult to diagnose – and even more likely to be overlooked – in people with cognitive and communicative difficulties.

4 **The masquerades**: represent conditions that may present as other problems or physical states. The most common of these are depression, diabetes mellitus, the adverse effects of medication, anaemia, thyroid disease, spinal dysfunction and urinary tract infections. All can potentially result in behavioural change in a person with intellectual disability. Some conditions (such as sleep apnoea in people with Down syndrome) should be considered in this context.

NATURE AND CONTEXT OF THE BEHAVIOUR
Finally, the nature and context of the challenging behaviour should be considered, and whether it communicates something about a particular medical problem (e.g. agitation at meal times might be an indication of difficulty swallowing, inhalation or reflux). Some of the autism spectrum disorders are associated with extreme pain tolerance so a thorough medical examination is important to identify injuries that may result from, or be causing, the behaviour.

Psychiatric assessment

Challenging behaviours may be related to psychiatric disorders which occur more commonly in people with intellectual disability (*see* Chapter 14, 'Assessment of Psychiatric Disorders', p. 111). While there may also be environmental and social causes for the behaviour, an accurate diagnosis of the psychiatric disorder or the challenging behaviour, and appropriate treatment, is often critical to managing the behaviour effectively. Depression and anxiety are much more common than psychotic disorders; they may present as challenging behaviours but be misinterpreted as psychotic symptoms. Autism spectrum disorders often coexist with intellectual disability and may be unrecognised; they can contribute to the development of challenging behaviour and impact on their management. *See* Chapter 26, 'Autism Spectrum Conditions' (p. 211).

Continued information gathering

It is good practice to collect information about the challenging behaviour during an assessment period, while working on a particular hypothesis and when implementing a treatment plan; this can include information from other involved individuals. Neglecting to collect information is the most common explanation for confusion regarding improvement of a situation, efficacy of an intervention or the 'true' cause of challenging behaviour.

PATIENT INFORMATION FILES
Many agencies keep patient information files, and they may go back over many years. They may be bulky, somewhat disorganised or difficult to read, but they may contain valuable information. They are important to view.

EXISTING DATA
Information is routinely collected in many settings, examples of which include a record of *pro re nata* (prn – when necessary) medication use, staff injury claims, incident records, bowel charts and seizure records. Ask to see them or ask a support person to make a summary (e.g. in some settings, a graph demonstrating the usage frequency of a prn medication gives an indication of the frequency and severity of challenging behaviour).

CHARTS
Charts are the most economical way for ongoing information to be collected. They need to be simple, and easy to use and interpret. Sleep pattern, weight changes and mood fluctuations are the most important indicators of well-being, and individual behaviours can be simply tracked across time by using a format similar to Table 12.4.

TABLE 12.4 Example of tracked behaviour over a week*

Behaviour	Date							Weekly total
	3 May	4 May	5 May	6 May	7 May	8 May	9 May	
Hits or kicks others	2	1	2	1	0	2	2	10
Screams	0	2	1	2	1	2	2	10
Steals food	1	2	0	1	0	1	1	6
Obsessed with one activity	2	0	2	2	1	0	0	7
Withdrawn	2	2	1	1	2	2	2	12
Daily total	7	7	6	7	4	7	7	

Key 0 = not a problem today; 1 = somewhat of a problem today; 2 = major problem today
* Based on the DBC-M ©, a daily behaviour monitoring system for people with developmental disability. The DBC-M chart and instructions are available as a supplement to the DBC scoring software manual. *See* www.med.monash.edu.au/spppm/research/devpsych/dbc.html for more information on the DBC.

5 Integrate other resources and assessments
Challenging behaviours are sometimes present for much of the life of the person with intellectual disability, and have probably been assessed previously by other professionals. These assessments may come from a range of sources (schools, speech

pathologists, psychologists, paediatricians) and can provide useful information to the clinician.

Services for people with intellectual disability may include management and assessment teams for changing challenging behaviours. These teams often use applied behaviour analysis (ABA) methodology that uses observational and experimental strategies to identify a 'function' that reinforces the behaviour. The team uses this information to develop a comprehensive behaviour intervention plan that may include five categories of potential intervention strategies to target:

➤ the ecological or setting event
➤ the immediate antecedent event
➤ the response and skill training
➤ the consequences of the behaviour
➤ emergency procedures.

These teams often recognise the need for medical assessment and may initiate a medical referral.

This information needs to be integrated with the clinician's own information before discussing the clinician's role in any ongoing management plan. If the underlying cause of the challenging behaviour is seen to be mainly medical, it might be appropriate for the medical practitioner to negotiate the lead role; however, if the challenging behaviour is seen as mainly a learnt behaviour, a behaviour management team or psychologist may have the lead role. Establishing links between the various professionals involved is important for both a thorough assessment and effective management.

6 Review and plan intervention

After making a comprehensive assessment (*see* 'Medical and psychiatric assessment and continued information gathering', p. 96), the clinician is in a position to review all available information and make a differential diagnosis as to the most likely cause of the challenging behaviour, and identify the factors contributing to it. This information includes a description of the challenging behaviour, the carer's concerns, the safety issues, medical and psychiatric problems and the objective measures about the behaviour and the person's well-being. The clinician should also have knowledge of the service system that provides for the person with intellectual disability. With all this at hand the most effective management plan can be discussed and formulated.

7 Manage and refer

Deciding on the most appropriate management strategies and referral options requires careful consideration of the potential benefits and risks of each option, the availability of resources and the long- and short-term effects on the person with intellectual disability. In general, assessment of more specialised medical and psychiatric problems requires referral to the appropriate specialist. Common general practice problems (such as depression or dysmenorrhoea) can be managed by the GP. Resources to manage the challenging behaviours may vary depending on the availability of local supports and the configuration of service systems. Whatever management strategy is decided on, it is important to maintain communication across the service providers and professionals involved; establishing these links is a critical part of the management process.

The management of challenging behaviour can also be assisted by educational and skill development, as well as modifications to the environment.

Educational and skill development

Educational and skill development assist a person with disability to learn new ways to interact more appropriately with others (e.g. social skills training and learning new skills to increase the person's opportunities). Increasing a person's competencies has a beneficial effect on self-esteem, as well as on the capacity to cope.

Environmental modifications

Environments in which effective and interactive communications can occur are essential. Appropriate living conditions, vocational opportunities, supportive social networks and meaningful leisure time are also important environmental provisions to maintain mental health for everyone.

Common problems for people with intellectual disability are:
➤ overstimulating and understimulating environments
➤ confusing or inconsistent communications to the person
➤ social isolation
➤ excessively demanding situations or expectations.

The person is likely to respond best to appropriate modifications to the environment, thus avoiding medication. For example, people who have a strong need for a predictable environment will respond well to a structured and consistent environment.

The individual, friends, family or staff can be referred to a specialist (e.g. speech therapist, psychologist) for advice regarding personalised communication strategies and augmented techniques (e.g. signing, visual diary).

8 Monitor and review

Once the diagnosis is made and the management plan established, it is important to regularly review the progress of the individual in terms of both the efficacy of the intervention strategy and the resilience of the diagnosis. The response to the intervention, and observations made over time, might open up the possibility of a new diagnosis and a more effective intervention strategy. Continuing the data collection strategies is, therefore, highly desirable.

FURTHER READING

- Einfeld SL, Tonge BJ. *Manual for the Developmental Behaviour Checklist (DBC)*. 2nd ed. Melbourne: School of Psychiatry, University of New South Wales, and Centre of Developmental Psychiatry, Monash University; 2002.
- Emerson E. *Challenging Behaviour: analysis and intervention with people with learning difficulties*. Cambridge: Cambridge University Press; 1995.
- Emerson E, Cummings R, Barrett S, *et al.* Challenging behaviour and community services 2. Who are the people who challenge the services? *Mental Handicap.* 1988; **16**: 16–19.
- Gourash LF. Assessing and managing medical factors. In: Barrett RP, editor. *Severe Behavior Disorders in the Mentally Retarded: non-drug approaches to treatment*. New York: Plenum Press; 1986, pp. 157–205.

- Murtagh J. A safe diagnostic strategy. In: Murtagh J. *General Practice*. 3rd ed. Sydney: McGraw-Hill; 2003, pp. 157–63.
- Ryan R, Sunada K. Medical evaluation of persons with mental retardation referred for psychiatric assessment. *Gen Hosp Psychiatry*. 1997; **19**(4): 274–80.
- Sovner R, Lowry MA. A behavioural methodology for diagnosing affective disorders in individuals with mental retardation. *The Habilitative Mental Healthcare Newsletter*. 1990; **9**(7): 55–61.

CHAPTER 13

Medication and challenging behaviour

Medical practitioners are often asked to make decisions about initiation, change or continuation of psychotropic medication to manage challenging behaviour in people with intellectual disability; however, the evidence base for such practice is limited. Additionally, ethical concerns arise when medication is used for behaviour that is underpinned by environmental rather than biological factors. Challenging behaviour has many determinants; unless the person is, or others are at risk, the cause of the challenging behaviour should be determined before prescribing psychotropic medications (*see* Chapter 12, 'Challenging Behaviour', p. 93). Medical and psychiatric disorders need to be identified and appropriately treated. For further information, *see* Chapter 14, 'Assessment of Psychiatric Disorders' (p. 111) and Chapter 15, 'Management of Psychiatric Disorders' (p. 121).

This chapter covers the principles of using psychotropic medication in people with intellectual disability and behavioural disturbance.

BEFORE PRESCRIBING MEDICATION

Many people with intellectual disability are on high doses and/or multiple medications without a clear rationale. Before any psychotropic medication is prescribed to manage challenging behaviour, a number of questions should be asked; *see* Box 13.1.

BOX 13.1 Questions to ask before prescribing psychotropic medication to manage challenging behaviour

1 Is the person – or are others – at risk of injury or harm because of the behavioural disturbance?
2 Has there been an assessment of the potential causes of the challenging behaviour?
3 What is your hypothesis regarding the behaviour?
4 What interventions have been tried and what were the outcomes?

> 5 Does the behaviour warrant treatment with medication without a clear psychiatric or medical diagnosis?
> 6 Is there a medication that may benefit this person with this behaviour?
> 7 Do the benefits outweigh the risks of prescribing this medication?
> 8 How will you monitor efficacy and adverse effects?

1 Is the person – or are others – at risk of injury or harm because of the behavioural disturbance?

Ensuring the safety of the person and others is vital. In acute situations, medication may be required to settle the person when they – or others – are at risk of serious harm or injury. Following drug administration, an assessment of the cause of the behaviour needs to be made.

2 Has there been an assessment of the potential causes of the challenging behaviour? and 3 What is your hypothesis regarding the behaviour?

The onset or exacerbation of challenging behaviour may be due to a myriad of causes including communication impairment, physical disorders that cause pain and discomfort, medication, medical and psychiatric disorders, and changes in the person's routine and their physical and social environment. Certain behaviour may be associated with particular syndromes (i.e. behavioural phenotypes); for example, skin picking is associated with a number of syndromes. However, exacerbation of typical behaviours still needs to be investigated and not simply ascribed to the syndrome. For further information, see Chapter 12, 'Challenging Behaviour' (p. 93), Chapter 14, 'Assessment of Psychiatric Disorders' (p. 111) and Chapter 8, 'Adult Healthcare' (p. 56).

4 What interventions have been tried and what were the outcomes?

What interventions have already been tried? Have changes have been made to the person's circumstances (e.g. more appropriate day placement)? Are communication strategies in place? Are behaviour management strategies being correctly implemented? How effective were the interventions? Are medications already prescribed to control challenging behaviour? Were there any adverse effects? Medications themselves may be the cause of the behavioural disturbance, and reducing or stopping medications may actually result in a positive outcome.

5 Does the behaviour warrant treatment with medication without a clear psychiatric or medical diagnosis?

What are the consequences of the behaviour for the person and for others? Is the behaviour of a frequency or severity great enough to warrant medication? Could the behaviour be managed without medication?

Medication may be justified to manage behaviour that:
➤ is ongoing
➤ may result in injury to the person – or others
➤ compromises the person's health and well-being
➤ distresses the person

➤ results in residential and day placement breakdown or other restrictions on the person's activities and community access.

6 Is there a medication that may benefit this person with this behaviour?

Certain psychotropic medications may be beneficial for particular types of problem behaviours. Psychotropic medication may enable the patient to make better use of a non-pharmacological approach (e.g. by lifting mood or reducing agitation with medication, the patient is better able to carry out relaxation techniques). However, psychotropic medications may also interfere with new learning and therefore complicate treatment. Treatment of behavioural emergencies, repeated and serious aggression, harmful self-injurious behaviour, continued agitated and restless behaviour, and stereotyped behaviours are discussed later in this chapter.

7 Do the benefits outweigh the risks of prescribing this medication?

People with intellectual disability have a higher prevalence of serious adverse effects with psychotropic medication than the rest of the population. The physician and those involved in medication supervision need to be continually aware of both the therapeutic and detrimental effects of these drugs in this population. Adverse effects of psychotropic medications in people with intellectual disability are discussed under 'Precautions in prescribing psychotropic medications' (p. 106).

8 How will you monitor efficacy and adverse effects?

Family and formal caregivers are not generally trained in the management of the sedated patient and should not be given this responsibility. Aspiration pneumonia is a leading cause of death in people with intellectual disability. Longer term use of psychotropic medication to manage challenging behaviour requires regular monitoring for efficacy and adverse effects. The monitoring of medications such as lithium can be problematic.

ESTABLISHING A TREATMENT PLAN

After assessment for psychiatric, physical, medical, iatrogenic and environmental aetiology, the physician – in consultation with the person (where possible), families and other support persons – should establish a treatment plan and define clear outcomes using the following steps.
➤ Define the target behaviour and outline techniques for measuring the behaviour.
➤ Take a reliable measure of the baseline behaviour.
➤ Formulate a hypothesis for the cause of the behaviour.
➤ Develop a treatment rationale – this may include a decision to reduce or cease current psychotropic medication.
➤ Assess the best available evidence for the impact of the medication on the target behaviour.
➤ Ensure the medication selected is the best choice for this person with this problem.
➤ Ensure that the potential benefits of the medication outweigh the potential risks.

➤ Define clear treatment outcomes.
➤ Ensure there are sufficient resources for reliable monitoring of the frequency and severity of the person's behaviour.
➤ Ensure that the efficacy and adverse effects of the medication can be adequately monitored.
➤ Develop a regular review process based on predetermined outcomes; this must be agreed to by all.
➤ Ensure that the person (and/or their legal guardian or support person) is aware of the potential benefits and adverse effects.
➤ Obtain consent from the person (or their legal guardian or support person).
➤ Start with a low dose; review the patient before dose increases and use the lowest effective dose.
➤ Base continuing treatment on response to, and adverse effects of, medication.
➤ Maintain a process for ongoing review.

The process of assessing the efficacy of a particular medication is a dynamic one. Assessment is dependent on the accuracy and reliability of both the definition of the behaviour and the observation techniques. In many cases, a clinician will find that it is not possible to satisfy all of the steps above. The question of how to proceed in such a situation depends on a risk–benefit analysis. Engaging the expertise of a psychiatrist, psychologist, or preferably a multidisciplinary team skilled in this area may be necessary. Pressure to begin, or increase or include, another medication – rather than training and supporting care staff – should be resisted.

A more detailed discussion of the relevant ethical issues may be found in Brown P. Ethical aspects of drug treatment. In: Bloch S, Chodoff P, editors. *Psychiatric Ethics*. 2nd ed. Oxford: Oxford University Press; 1991.

PRECAUTIONS IN PRESCRIBING PSYCHOTROPIC MEDICATIONS

People with intellectual disability may have a range of comorbid conditions, physical congenital defects and neurodevelopmental brain abnormalities that can heighten sensitivity to medication. For example, people with Prader-Willi syndrome are usually of short stature, obese with a low lean muscle mass and hypotonia. They are at risk of respiratory failure; hence the use of benzodiazepines, especially parenterally, can be hazardous.

In addition, swallowing problems are common, especially in people with cerebral palsy. Airway protection may be compromised in sedated patients.

The cognitive and communicative impairments common to people with intellectual disability mean that adverse effects may be present but not reported or recognised. Behavioural change may be a form of communication that represents distress resulting from adverse effects of the medication, or the medication itself may be the cause of behavioural change. Antipsychotic medication – especially 'typical' antipsychotic drugs – may result in akathisia and dystonias. Antiepileptics may impair cognition and adversely affect behaviour. Treatment with benzodiazepines may result in paradoxical reactions through disinhibition.

Doses in this chapter are those recommended for adults. A general principle for the use of medications in people with intellectual disability is to 'start low and go slow'. For some people, it may be prudent to start at half the recommended dose. Whenever possible advice should be sought from a Consultant Psychiatrist for the

Intellectually Disabled and in the UK it would be unusual practice to prescribe medications other than those for acute disorders on a long-term basis without such advice probably as the result of a formal referral.

BEHAVIOURAL EMERGENCIES

Usually, the patient will settle spontaneously. Sometimes behavioural emergencies are triggered when a person is in an unfamiliar environment in frightening circumstances (e.g. hospital admission). It is important to consider the situation from the person's point of view, to ensure that efforts are made to alleviate anxiety and fear. Ensuring the safety of the patient and waiting until they have settled may be the best course of action; however, in some cases the level of danger may require the use of sedating medication before clearly defining a cause. Adequate monitoring of response and vital signs should be ensured. Once the patient settles, the clinician should reassess the situation and look for a situational, medical or psychiatric cause of the behaviour.

There is a scant evidence base regarding the safe doses of medications that can be used to manage behavioural emergencies in people with developmental disability. The upper limit doses of medications recommended in the BNF could prove excessive for some people with intellectual disability.

The care staff in community residential units are not nurses and they should not be asked to care for a heavily sedated person.

Respiratory complications are the major cause of premature death in people with intellectual disability. Monitoring of vital signs and protection of the airway by nursing or medical professionals is mandatory. The patient may need to be transferred to hospital for monitoring.

REPEATED AND SERIOUS ACTS OF AGGRESSION

Aggressive behaviours include physical aggression, verbal threats and abuse, and property destruction. Disorders such as mania need to be considered.

The continuing risk of aggressive behaviour to the person themselves and to those around them, and resistance to behaviour management programmes, may necessitate the use of medication. Diminishing the tendency to aggressive behaviours may allow environmental and behavioural interventions to be more effective.

Repeated and serious acts of aggression are often intermittent and due to poor impulse control following some provocation. Escalating the doses of medication is not usually efficacious and the use of short-term sedation may be more appropriate.

Beta-blockers

The beta-blockers have been demonstrated to moderate aggressive behaviour, particularly explosive–aggressive episodes. Beta-blockers, e.g. propranolol 80 to 280 mg orally, daily, are less likely to cause sedation than other medications.

Beta-blockers are contraindicated in patients with asthma or severe peripheral vascular disease and some patients with heart failure.

Lithium

There is probably more evidence that lithium moderates aggressive behaviour than any other medication. However, the narrow therapeutic range and the need for regular blood tests are factors that often limit its use. Lithium may be considered when aggression is associated with autistic tendencies and occurs with hyperactivity:

➤ lithium 250 mg orally, twice daily, increasing to therapeutic levels in increments of 250 mg at intervals ranging from three days to four weeks, depending on the clinical circumstance and blood levels.

Some patients need levels of 0.8 to 1 mmol/L before a response is seen. *See* Chapter 15, 'Management of Psychiatric Disorders' (p. 130) for details about the adverse effects and monitoring required.

Sodium valproate
The evidence base for the use of sodium valproate is limited; however, it is widely used and anecdotal reports suggest that it reduces mood instability and the tendency to impulsive action.

Dosing is related to the clinical response rather than to the serum levels:

➤ sodium valproate 100 mg orally, twice daily, increasing in increments of 100 mg at intervals ranging from one to four weeks, depending on the clinical circumstances and response to treatment.

For more information, *see* Chapter 15, 'Management of Psychiatric Disorders' (p. 131).

Carbamazepine
Available evidence suggests that the effect of carbamazepine is limited to its sedative properties. It has been known to cause aggressive behaviour and liver damage. It should no longer be used as a first-line drug:

➤ carbamazepine 100 to 200 mg orally, daily in two divided doses, initially, increasing weekly by increments of 100 mg per day, up to doses similar to those used in epilepsy.

Antipsychotic medications
The full range of antipsychotic medications – both typical and atypical – have been used to ameliorate aggressive behaviours. The choice of which antipsychotic to use is directed by the adverse effect profile, bearing in mind that people with disability often have problems with obesity, constipation, oral health and mobility. Even apparently low doses can result in considerable functional impairment.

Sometimes a combination of a mood stabiliser and low-dose risperidone (0.5 mg daily) or olanzapine (2.5 mg daily) together with a behaviour management programme is likely to be better tolerated and more effective than escalating doses of an antipsychotic. However, the potential for drug interactions needs to be considered.

Selective serotonin reuptake inhibitors
Depression is common and may present with irritable mood and associated aggressive behaviours; the diagnosis is often missed. Selective serotonin reuptake inhibitors (SSRIs) have been shown to moderate aggressive behaviour, sometimes without proven depressive symptomatology. A combination of antidepressant and anxiolytic effects may contribute to the efficacy of SSRIs. As SSRIs are well tolerated

and have relatively few adverse effects, a trial of therapy may be worthwhile. *See* Chapter 15, 'Management of Psychiatric Disorders' (p. 129) for adverse effects and monitoring.

People with intellectual disability appear to be more sensitive to SSRIs and may become agitated or manic. Commencing at half the standard recommended doses with half-dose increments is recommended.

HARMFUL SELF-INJURIOUS BEHAVIOUR

Self-injurious behaviour in people with intellectual disability can range from relatively harmless self-hitting and scratching to injuries resulting in major physical damage or even death. The severity of this behaviour and its resistance to behavioural management programmes has resulted in a range of medications being used for treatment.

Antipsychotics

Antipsychotic medications may have a role to play by reducing stereotypical self-injurious behaviours. The usual caveats regarding the use of these medications (as outlined previously) apply.

Naltrexone

Naltrexone is a narcotic antagonist. One theory for its use in this indication is that self-injurious behaviour is maintained in the individual by a build-up of endogenous opioids or beta endorphins that modulate pain and induce a feeling of euphoria. Its use should be restricted to patients with serious levels of self-injurious behaviour. In adults, use:

➤ naltrexone 50 mg orally, daily initially, increasing if necessary to a maximum dose of 1 to 2 mg/kg daily.

CONTINUED AGITATED AND RESTLESS BEHAVIOUR

If the person is taking an antipsychotic, consider the possibility of akathisia being the cause of agitated or restless behaviour.

Lithium

Lithium dosage and administration are similar to that used for aggressive behaviour (*see* p. 130).

Clomipramine

Clomipramine has been shown to be effective when the behaviour resembles obsessive-compulsive disorder. It has frequent anticholinergic adverse effects (e.g. sweating, hot flushes, tachycardia) that may be distressing to the patient. Drowsiness, confusion and disorientation may also be a problem. Use clomipramine 25 mg orally, at night, slowly increasing in increments of 25 mg every three days to 150 mg at night, depending on response or adverse effects. After four to six weeks, increase further if necessary at weekly intervals by increments of 25 to 50 mg per day, up to 300 mg at night.

Alternatively, an SSRI can be trialled to avoid the drowsiness and anticholinergic adverse effects of clomipramine.

Clonidine

Clonidine has been widely used and may be beneficial for the hyperactivity symptoms and concentration difficulties experienced by patients with fragile X syndrome. It has been used alone or in combination with dexamphetamine or methylphenidate. Clonidine has a tendency to sedate the patient and blood pressure should be monitored regularly. Sudden cessation should be avoided as rebound hypertension may occur. Use clonidine 50 micrograms orally, daily, increasing if necessary by 50 micrograms every third day up to a maximum of 4 micrograms/kg daily in one to three divided doses. Clonidine's duration of action lasts only two to four hours after oral administration. Recommended doses do not generally produce major problems with sedation or hypotension, provided the dose is increased slowly.

STEREOTYPED BEHAVIOUR

Stereotyped behaviour consists of repetitive, topographically invariant, motor acts that serve no adaptive function. Activities such as rocking the body, hand-flapping or head-rolling occur frequently in people with developmental disability. A number of large and methodologically sound studies have shown the antipsychotics – in particular low-dose risperidone – to be effective in decreasing stereotyped behaviour.

ESSENTIAL READING

- Deb S, Clarke D, Unwin G. *Using Medication to Manage Behaviour Problems among Adults with a Learning Disability. Quick Reference Guide.* University of Birmingham, MENCAP, The Royal College of Psychiatrists, London; 2006.

FURTHER READING

- Aman MG. Overview of pharmacotherapy: current status and future directions. *J Ment Defic Res.* 1987; **31**(2): 121–30.
- Baumeister AA, Todd ME, Sevin JA. Efficacy and specificity of pharmacological therapies for behavioral disorders in persons with mental retardation. *Clin Neuropharmacol.* 1993; **16**(4): 271–94.
- Luchins DJ, Dojka D. Lithium and propranolol in aggression and self-injurious behavior in the mentally retarded. *Psychopharmacol Bull.* 1989; **25**(3): 372–5.

CHAPTER 14

Assessment of psychiatric disorders

Psychiatric disorders in people with intellectual disability are two to three times more common than in the general population. Estimates of prevalence vary widely depending on sample selection, the definition of psychiatric disorder, which diagnostic criteria are used, and the skill and experience of the clinicians. There are many reasons for the higher prevalence of psychiatric disorder in some people with intellectual disability, including neurodevelopmental abnormalities, genetic factors, high rates of epilepsy and other comorbid conditions, personality development, cognitive impairment limiting capacity to cope with stress, and adverse social circumstances. Table 14.1 lists the risk factors for psychiatric disorder in people with intellectual disability.

TABLE 14.1 Risk factors for psychiatric disorder in people with intellectual disability

Biological	Underlying neurodevelopmental brain abnormalities
	Genetic disorders/behavioural phenotypes (e.g. fragile X syndrome)
	Family history of psychiatric disorder
	Epilepsy
	Comorbid medical conditions
	Medications
Psychological	Impaired social cognition
	Limited coping skills
	Limited control over life circumstances
	Repeated losses or separations
	Communication impairments
	Impaired acquisition of social, recreational and interpersonal skills
	Low self-esteem from failure, rejection and perceived unfavourable appearance
	Personality development
Social	Family functioning
	Lack of social support and social isolation
	Adverse life events including abuse
	Rejection, stigma, labelling and negative expectations
	Expressed emotion at home, community residential unit, workplace or day placement

PRESENTATION OF PSYCHIATRIC DISORDERS

The presentation of psychiatric disorders in people with mild intellectual disability and good communication skills is similar to that of the general population, and standard diagnostic criteria such as DSM-IV and ICD-10 can generally be used. However, the application of standard diagnostic criteria to people with more severe levels of intellectual disability and communication impairment is not valid – these criteria are reliant on a person being able to verbally self-report subjective experiences, and do not take into account the behavioural manifestations or atypical features of psychiatric disorder in people with intellectual disability.

The Royal College of Psychiatrists have published *DC-LD: Diagnostic criteria for psychiatric disorders, for use with adults with learning disabilities/mental retardation.* The DC-LD is based upon ICD-10, and provides consensus diagnostic criteria for psychiatric disorders in people with intellectual disability.

People with intellectual disability are often reliant on others for referral for psychiatric assessment. This means that people with challenging behaviours are likely to be referred, whereas someone who is quietly depressed may not be referred for assessment. There are few specialist psychiatric services for people with intellectual disability within Australia. Medical and mental health professionals receive little (if any) training in the assessment and management of psychiatric disorders in people with intellectual disability. Hence, psychiatric disorders in people with intellectual disability are often not diagnosed – or are misdiagnosed – and therefore not appropriately treated. When services specific to intellectual disability are not available, the GP's expertise and knowledge of the patient assumes greater significance.

ASSESSMENT

The most common problem a GP is asked to assess in a person with intellectual disability is challenging behaviour.

Challenging behaviour in a person with intellectual disability may be due to many reasons (e.g. pain or discomfort, medical illness, psychiatric disorder, communication impairment, reaction to circumstances). Challenging behaviour may be attributed to the intellectual disability alone, without sufficient attention being given to other possible causes. This practice has been called 'diagnostic overshadowing' and clinicians who are aware of it are least likely to practise it. An optimal assessment involves a bio-psychosocial approach by specially trained clinicians to identify all the possible physical and psychiatric factors, while being aware of the effect of environmental influences.

Multiple factors may be responsible for challenging behaviour presentation (*see* Chapter 12, 'Challenging Behaviour', p. 93). Consider any combination of factors. No factors are mutually exclusive.

History taking

History taking is the central part of a psychiatric assessment. In addition to the history of the presenting complaint, there may be a family history of intellectual disability or psychiatric problems. The developmental history may reveal the cause of the intellectual disability, temperamental and personality factors, autism spectrum disorders, level of functioning, education, and past medical and psychiatric assessments. It may not be possible to take a full history at a single appointment;

history taking may need to occur over a number of sessions. If the situation is acute, emergency psychiatric care should be sought.

Problems using informers

It is important to know the reason for referral for psychiatric assessment. The reasons vary depending upon the professional background, experience, attitudes and patient knowledge of the informant. Staff who attend medical appointments with their clients may not be in full possession of all the facts, and they may need help in identifying the most relevant information (*see* Chapter 2). Staff may sometimes bias the interview so that a doctor will alter medication in an effort to control difficult behaviours, and perhaps not appreciate the importance of a full assessment being performed. Some staff mistrust the medical profession and it requires patience, skill and tact to work with them. Recommendations to avoid informer bias are summarised in Box 14.1.

BOX 14.1 Recommendations to avoid informer bias

- Adopt a broad bio-psychosocial model of history taking and assessment so that all possibilities are considered.
- Obtain corroborative information and listen to all parties who may accompany the person with intellectual disability to the interview.
- Consider implementing the use of monitoring charts to increase the level of objective reporting (*see* Chapter 12, 'Challenging Behaviour', p. 99).
- Whenever possible, see the person with intellectual disability on their own for part of the interview. The patient may be less likely to experience subtle coercion or pressure when interviewed alone, and will be able to detail problems and issues from a personal perspective. This is an essential component of the psychiatric assessment.

Response consistency and validity

When interviewing a person with intellectual disability, it is vital to ascertain that the answers provided are consistent and valid. To improve response reliability, consider the following.

➤ Start by asking questions to which the patient can confidently give correct answers. Try to establish rapport and decrease the anxiety of the patient.
➤ Use an 'anchor event' (e.g. a recent clearly identifiable and memorable event such as a recent birthday or the last Christmas) to help assess subjective duration of symptoms and test memory function.
➤ Ask the same question in different ways or at different times in the interview.
➤ Beware of adopting an approach that leads the patient to respond affirmatively to every enquiry. Indirect or open-ended questions sometimes provide more reliable responses.

Communication impairments and sensory deficits

Communication impairments can affect how a person recounts feelings and experiences. People with sensory deficits may use sign language and/or interpreters and recall may become biased or distorted. Aim to establish an adequate and reliable method of communication in each individual circumstance.

In people with severe communication impairments, psychiatric diagnosis may be made on the basis of observed signs and behaviours only. Standard diagnostic criteria need to be translated into observable criteria, including behavioural equivalents. An example of this situation is a person who may not be able to state that they feel depressed but appears sad, may not smile or laugh and may cry often. Support persons can observe and document the frequency, duration, setting and severity of relevant behaviours.

See Chapter 12, 'Challenging Behaviour' (p. 95) for a discussion on behavioural equivalents and further examples of behavioural equivalents, and other observable features of depression, hypomania and mania.

Other assessment factors

Dr Robert Sovner highlights common sources of diagnostic error in the assessment of challenging behaviour in people with intellectual disability:

INTELLECTUAL DISTORTION

Concrete thinking and impaired communication leads/causes the person with intellectual disability to be unable to label their own inner experiences and report on them.

For example, a woman with intellectual disability and episodic severe self-injury repeated over and over 'a man in black, a man in black'. She was never able to further explain the significance of this phrase.

PSYCHOSOCIAL MASKING

Impoverished social skills and life experiences can make a person with intellectual disability be judged as very unsophisticated; key symptoms can be missed and diagnostic errors may result.

For example, a man living in supported accommodation episodically spent his pocket money at a charity shop on grey trousers, white shirts and business ties which he wore while attempting to do tasks normally done by staff. He initially was quite helpful, but soon became annoying and intrusive, and when reprimanded, laughed uproariously and swore copiously. His hypomanic episodes over many years had not been diagnosed.

COGNITIVE DISINTEGRATION

When a person with intellectual disability is under stress, they may experience a greater than usual disruption in information processing, and consequently present in a very bizarre and psychotic state. A misdiagnosis of schizophrenia may result.

For example, a young man with mild intellectual disability was unexpectedly sacked from his job. He began to tremble, could not speak and ran off sobbing wildly. His parents found him hours later wandering dazed and confused, unable to describe where he had been or what had happened. He remained disturbed, mumbling to himself and unable to do simple tasks for several days.

BASELINE EXAGGERATION

A person with cognitive deficits may experience an increase in the frequency, duration or severity of pre-existing challenging behaviours. Careful attention in an assessment is needed to tease this out, as important diagnostic information can be easily overlooked.

For example, a man with moderate intellectual disability often paced around and, at times, wandered off. Over a period of a few weeks his pacing became faster; when staff intervened he ran away and was retrieved by police a long way from his residence. In addition, he was not sleeping well and had made sexual advances to female staff.

Examinations and investigations

For those presenting with challenging behaviour or a suspected psychiatric disorder, the following investigations are a mandatory part of the psychiatric assessment:

➤ full psychiatric history taking (including family and developmental history)
➤ mental state examination
➤ thorough physical examination
➤ haematological, biochemical and endocrine screening.

Where a diagnosis of epilepsy is suspected, an electroencephalogram (EEG) is essential. Other brain imaging techniques and a neurological opinion may be indicated, and are particularly relevant where focal signs exist.

ANXIETY DISORDERS

Anxiety disorders are common both in the general population and in people with intellectual disability. All anxiety disorders can produce significant levels of functional disability and handicap.

Generalised anxiety disorder and panic disorder

The anxiety and worry associated with generalised anxiety disorder may be expressed as fear and doubts about the present, the future, personal health and the welfare of significant others. Associated features include repetitive questioning, restlessness, agitation, aggression, and sleep and concentration problems. Panic attacks may occur and, if frequent, may warrant a separate diagnosis of panic disorder.

Obsessive-compulsive disorder

Obsessive-compulsive disorder may present in a person with mild intellectual disability as recurring, intrusive and distressing thoughts (obsessions) associated with anxiety. This may lead to repetitive acts (compulsions) to allay the fears and consequences associated with the obsessions. In people with intellectual disability, obsessions are usually less prominent, and compulsions alone may be the predominant symptom. It may be difficult to distinguish between compulsions and the stereotypic and ritualistic behaviours of autism.

Phobias

Simple phobias are common and, if causing significant disturbance in function, may require desensitisation procedures.

Social phobia is difficult to diagnose in people with intellectual disability, as many of the manifestations can overlap with the features of the intellectual disability and autistic spectrum disorders, or be a consequence of the lack of education and socialisation.

MOOD DISORDERS
Depression

The diagnosis of depression requires a two-week period (at least) of depressed mood, loss of interest or pleasure and associated symptoms. People with mild/moderate intellectual disability may express a wish to die and may even attempt suicide. People with greater degrees of intellectual disability may not be able to tell others they are feeling depressed. However, depressed mood may manifest itself by the person crying, having restricted affect, smiling less and losing their humour. Depression may also present with irritable mood.

Other disorders (e.g. hypomania) may also present with irritable mood, so other indicators of depression need to be identified (e.g. loss of interest and loss of energy) which may manifest as the person not wanting to get out of bed to go to day placement, needing prompting to carry out their assigned chores, or no longer doing things that they enjoy (e.g. watching television and videos, looking at magazines or listening to music). There are usually coexisting changes in sleep, appetite and weight, plus psychomotor agitation or retardation. Other observable associated features may include regression in skills; loss of enjoyment of, interest in, or refusal to, participate in usual activities; social withdrawal; diminished communication; increased anxiety; and more general behavioural disturbance (including verbal or physical aggression or self-injurious behaviours).

Table 14.2 documents common observable features of depression in people with intellectual disability.

For example, a 28-year-old woman with a history of minor skin picking presents with a two-month history of severe self-injury with open wounds on her arms and legs. Over this time she has been irritable, unhappy and has been found crying in her room. She hits staff when they try to get her into the bus in the morning. She needs lots of encouragement to help with the evening chores, picks at her food and goes to her room rather than watch her favourite television shows with her housemates. She no longer joins in conversations and shrugs when staff try to talk with her. Night staff have sometimes found her sitting alone in the lounge room in the dark.

Bipolar affective disorder

Bipolar affective disorder may present with recurring depressive episodes (see above) interspersed with hypomanic or manic episodes. In a hypomanic episode there may be extreme irritability, as well as indications of elevated mood (e.g. inappropriate laughter, singing, whistling, skipping). Activity levels may be greatly increased and have a 'driven' quality. The person may become extremely hyperactive, disorganised, destructive of property (e.g. hurling of furniture) or physically aggressive towards others. Talk can be loud and incessant, jumping between topics that have grandiose content. In people who are non-verbal, there may be an increased amount and volume of vocalisations (including shouting). In people with intellectual disability, grandiosity may involve wanting to do things that are out of proportion to the person's skills and abilities (e.g. driving a car, getting married and raising a family); *see* the section on psychosocial masking (p. 114). In mania, the dysfunction is more severe and may be accompanied by mood-congruent delusions and hallucinations.

For example, a 40-year-old man with idiopathic intellectual disability repeatedly

TABLE 14.2 Features of depression in adults with intellectual disability

Behaviour	Observable features
Depressed mood	Tearfulness Appears sad Less or no smiling Less or no laughing
Irritable mood	Short temper Verbal aggression Physical aggression Property damage
Loss of interest or pleasure	Refusing to, or needing prompting to, participate in routine activities No longer watching or enjoying favourite TV shows Unable to be cheered up
Increased anxiety	Seeking reassurance Repetitive questioning Increase in repetitive behaviours
Associated features	Spending more time alone Talking to, or interacting with, others less Loss of skills No longer completing tasks Self-injurious behaviour

Biological symptoms	Change in sleep pattern:
	  getting up during the night
	  getting up early
	  difficult to wake up in the morning
	Eating more or less
	Loss or increase in weight
	Psychomotor agitation or retardation

Baseline exaggeration of pre-existing behaviours	

absconds at night from his community residence. A review of his files shows that this has been a recurrent pattern of behaviour since he was 17 years old. At these times, and on this occasion, he is noted to be 'silly', giggling inappropriately, hyperactive, going without sleep for two to three days at a time. He masturbates in the lounge room, intrudes into other people's bedrooms, turns the lights on and off, plays his stereo at full volume and yells, shouts and sings. He is also irritable, physically threatening and, at times, aggressive to others. He has hurled furniture and torn down curtains and blinds.

See Table 14.3 for behaviour and observable features of hypomania and mania.

Mixed mood episode
Mixed mood episodes are not uncommon in people with intellectual disability. Mood is likely to be irritable and labile. In some instances, agitated depression (with

TABLE 14.3 Behaviour and observable features of hypomania and mania

Behaviour	Observable features
Elevated mood	• Extreme happiness, cheerfulness • Inappropriate laughing, singing, whistling
Irritable mood	• Verbal aggression • Physical aggression • Property destruction
Biological features	• Sleeping less (may not sleep for days) • Weight loss or gain • Psychomotor agitation
Associated behaviours	• Increased intensity and frequency of usual activities or traits (e.g. eating, drinking coffee, smoking) • Changing from one activity to another • Increased activity levels (including pacing, walking long distances, rearranging or throwing furniture) • Increased amount, volume and pressure of speech or vocalisations • 'Cockiness', not responding to usual instructions and redirections • 'Colourful' dress, wearing best clothes to day placement or wearing more jewellery • Disinhibited behaviour (including sexual disinhibition)

markedly irritable mood) may be difficult to distinguish from hypomania. Hence, it is crucial to identify mood congruent features.

PSYCHOSES

Psychoses of whatever type are characterised by loss of touch with reality – as manifested by the presence of delusions, hallucinations or disorganisation in thought patterns and behaviour. In people with intellectual disability, wishful thinking (fantasies) must be distinguished from true delusions (fixed, false, immovable beliefs that are out of keeping with the person's circumstances, education and background). Self-talk may also be misinterpreted as a response to auditory hallucinations.

Schizophrenia may be extremely difficult to diagnose when a patient's IQ is below 50, or if they are mute or unable to express themself in any way. Withdrawal, isolation, regression in skills and function, fear and inexplicable targeting of another person may be seen in combination with bizarre and disorganised behaviours. Catatonic features appear to be more common in people with intellectual disability than in the general population.

The elucidation of psychotic symptoms requires skill. Formal thought disorder appears to be less florid. Abnormal use of language (pragmatic language disorders) seen in autistic spectrum disorders or fragile X syndrome may be mistaken for thought disorder. Delusions and hallucinations tend to be more simple in theme and content (psychosocial masking) than the more complex delusions and auditory hallucinations seen in people without intellectual disability (e.g. persecutory delusions may relate to others trying to get the person into trouble, rather than elaborate involvement of police and spy agencies). Beware of asking whether the person hears voices, as this will generate a high false-positive response.

Caution is required so that self-talk and fantasy are not diagnosed as psychotic symptoms.

COMORBIDITIES

Many medical problems are either unrecognised or poorly managed, and may contribute to a psychiatric disorder. Comorbidities not only affect the presentation of psychiatric problems but also compound difficulties in assessment and management.

Comorbidities are frequent and include epilepsy, cerebral damage, autism, sensory deficits, medical disorders, medication effects, chronic pain and behavioural disorders. They render the process of labelling a presenting problem as exclusively psychiatric more difficult in people with intellectual disability.

Epilepsy

Epilepsy may produce psychiatric symptomatology in the pre-ictal, ictal, postictal and interictal stages (e.g. the interictal affect-preserved paranoid psychosis seen in people who have complex partial seizures). It may result in delirium states with agitation and aggression, and these may be confused with behavioural problems. Nocturnal seizures may go undetected and may present as early morning behavioural problems or bedwetting.

Of more controversy is the 'epileptic personality' that has been described in people with complex partial seizures and often those with a past history of institutional care. In this condition, personality traits of rigidity and obsessionality, hypergraphia, circumstantiality, inabilities to shift idea sets and cross-dressing have been described.

Pseudoseizures are not uncommon in people with intellectual disability; they may be associated with actually having epilepsy, living with other people with epilepsy, illness behaviour or personality problems.

Autism spectrum disorders

Autism spectrum disorders (pervasive developmental disorders) may present a range of bizarre and bewildering behaviours. Autism spectrum disorders may be comorbid with psychiatric disorder or other medical problems – in particular, epilepsy. Carers and clinicians may be alerted to the possibility of another psychiatric or medical illness by a combination of an alteration in functioning, the development of new symptoms or the exacerbation of pre-existing behaviours. Many people with intellectual disability may have autistic traits that have not previously been identified and may underpin the disturbance in behaviour. Hence, when assessing a person with intellectual disability and challenging behaviour, it is important to take a thorough developmental history.

Impairments in prefrontal function

Abnormalities of prefrontal and subcortical circuits can result in a range of cognitive, behavioural and psychiatric symptoms. Impairments in executive functions (dorsolateral prefrontal cortex) may manifest as problems with planning, initiating and completing tasks without structure and guidance; and inability to cope with change and novel situations. Medial prefrontal abnormalities may result in apathy and amotivation while orbital prefrontal abnormalities can present with disinhibited and impulsive behaviours; emotional lability, exaggerated emotional responses and aggressive behaviour; and poor social judgement. Impairments in prefrontal functioning can result in greater levels of disability than would be expected for a given IQ, and the inability to cope with the flux of life may lead to episodic severe challenging behaviour.

FURTHER READING

- Davis JP, Judd FK, Herrman H. Depression in adults with intellectual disability. Part 1: a review. *Aust N Z J Psychiatry.* 1997; **31**(2): 232–42.
- Davis JP, Judd FK, Herrman H. Depression in adults with intellectual disability. Part 2: a pilot study. *Aust N Z J Psychiatry.* 1997; **31**(2): 243–51.
- Einfeld SL. Clinical assessment of psychiatric symptoms in mentally retarded individuals. *Aust N Z J Psychiatry.* 1992; **26**(1): 48–63.
- Royal College of Psychiatrists. *DC-LD: Diagnostic criteria for psychiatric disorders for use with adults with learning disabilities/mental retardation.* London: Gaskell; 2001.
- Sovner R. Limiting factors in the use of DSM-III criteria with mentally ill/mentally retarded persons. *Psychopharmacol Bull.* 1986; **22**(4): 1055–9.

CHAPTER 15

Management of psychiatric disorders

The management of psychiatric disorders in people with intellectual disability follows the same bio-psychosocial principles as those applied in the general population.

This chapter focuses on issues of particular relevance to caring for people with intellectual disability and psychiatric disorders and in general should be undertaken within a shared care system between primary care and the consultant led team of psychiatry for those with intellectual disability.

KEY MANAGEMENT POINTS

The management of psychiatric disorders involves psychosocial and pharmacological approaches in individually tailored combinations. Less serious psychiatric disorders can be managed with regular consultations, and with the involvement of families, other support persons and relevant services, depending on the social and support needs of the person. Family and other support persons can assist with diagnosis and monitoring of treatment response by keeping charts and diaries of symptoms and behaviours.

Challenging behaviours may coexist with a psychiatric disorder – pre-existing behaviours may become exaggerated or new behaviours may be learned as a consequence of the psychiatric disorder. Psychiatric and behavioural treatments may need to be combined.

However, for acute psychiatric disorders such as psychotic or manic episodes, or depressive episodes complicated by suicide risk or inadequate oral intake, more intensive psychiatric care is required. People with intellectual disability may be vulnerable in acute inpatient units; management may be more appropriate in their home environment with support from the local community psychiatric team.

Community residential units are homes and should not be viewed as psychiatric inpatient units. The impact on the other residents of living with someone who has an acute psychiatric disorder needs to be taken into consideration. Care staff provide day-to-day care and may not be on active duty overnight. They are not healthcare professionals and are not trained to undertake nursing duties such as monitoring mental state, which is the responsibility of the treating medical practitioner or mental health team. Care staff should be given instructions in writing about when to use medications prn or when to seek an unscheduled review.

Regulations regarding prn medications vary depending on local practice and the attitude of staff and management.

Admission to a psychiatric unit may be indicated when:

➤ the person or others are at risk of serious harm

➤ management may require regular monitoring of mental state, prn medication or seclusion

➤ treatments such as electroconvulsive therapy are indicated.

PSYCHOLOGICAL INTERVENTIONS
Supportive psychotherapies

The components of supportive psychotherapy include empathic listening, education, assistance with problem solving, encouragement and (when appropriate) reassurance. Education and problem solving need to be appropriate to the person's language development. The use of stories and pictures (such as the *Books Beyond Words* series available through the Royal College of Psychiatrists) are useful.

Behavioural therapies

Behavioural therapies are commonly used as effective treatments for behavioural problems. They may have a place in the treatment of psychiatric disorders where the psychiatric symptoms (e.g. aggression or non-participation in usual activities as a symptom of depressive disorder) have become reinforced by social or environmental factors (e.g. support person response).

Cognitive behavioural therapy

Cognitive behavioural therapy (CBT) is a form of psychotherapy that involves techniques to change cognition and behaviour that may be causing or maintaining inappropriate emotion. It uses a combination of many cognitive and behavioural elements for understanding and treating patients.

The therapeutic alliance is very important for cognitive behavioural therapy in people with intellectual disability, as it is with the general population. However, it may take a long time to form a relationship conducive to cognitive behavioural therapy. People with intellectual disability may have had lifelong experiences of rejection, failed intervention and adverse experiences with caregivers; they may have been referred for treatment of proscribed behaviour (i.e. they think they are 'in trouble'). These factors all negatively impact on the relationship with the therapist.

Psychoanalytically oriented psychotherapy

The use of psychoanalytically oriented psychotherapy in people with intellectual disability has a long tradition; however, there is a dearth of evidence in the research literature about its use. People with intellectual disability face the same life crises and hurdles as people in general; cognitive impairment, including impairments in social cognition and other developmental factors, may create further complexities in resolving these issues.

PHARMACOLOGICAL MANAGEMENT
Principles of psychotropic medication use

Psychotropic medication should only be prescribed for:

➤ a diagnosed psychiatric disorder

➤ a therapeutic trial for a suspected psychiatric disorder
➤ challenging behaviour under the certain circumstances described in
  Chapter 13, 'Medication and Challenging Behaviour' (p. 103).

Indications for the continuing prescription of psychotropic medications need to be regularly reviewed. Antipsychotic medications, in particular, are widely prescribed in people with intellectual disability without a clear diagnostic formulation or management plan. The diagnosis of psychotic disorders is more difficult to make reliably in people with intellectual disability and tends to be overdiagnosed. Mood disorders, however, are frequently misdiagnosed as either a psychotic disorder or as challenging behaviour. Escalating doses of an antipsychotic medication is unlikely to resolve a manic episode (which requires mood stabilisation) or a depressive episode for which antidepressant medication is indicated. Diagnosis of psychiatric disorders is discussed in Chapter 14, 'Assessment of Psychiatric Disorders' (p. 111). It is reasonable to seek expert opinion if you are unsure of the diagnosis or where there is poor response to treatment.

Principles of prescribing psychotropic medications for people with intellectual disability are outlined in Box 15.1. Pharmacological treatment of psychiatric disorders in people with intellectual disability is in essence no different than the treatment of the same disorders in the general population. Often, people with intellectual disability are sensitive to the behavioural, cognitive and physical adverse effects of psychotropic medications. The increase in challenging behaviour resulting from the medication may be misinterpreted as evidence of a need to increase the medication, thus setting up a cycle of escalating disturbance prompting dosage increases. The antipsychotics and benzodiazepines are particularly prone to producing this problem. Antipsychotic medications – both typical and atypical – can cause significant psychomotor retardation that may result in functional decline or be mistaken for depression. Treatment with antidepressant medications may result in a manic switch. Most antipsychotics and antidepressants can increase the seizure frequency of patients with epilepsy.

BOX 15.1 Key points to observe when using psychotropic medication

- Obtain consent before prescribing.
- Prescribe medication at low doses (initially) and increase the dose gradually.
- Review the type, dose and route of administration of antipsychotics regularly, also the therapeutic and adverse effects.
- Consider changing a person on a typical antipsychotic to an atypical antipsychotic – especially if there are significant adverse effects or limited efficacy.
- Determine the length of trial to be pursued at the start of treatment, so that medication can be withdrawn after the trial period if it is not effective.
- Consider the use of depot antipsychotics when compliance is a problem (provided adverse effects can be monitored adequately).
- Review the use of depot antipsychotics if compliance with oral treatment is not a problem.
- Set clear review dates.

- Establish a reliable method of monitoring treatment response (e.g. a daily chart of the number of incidents of a specified type).
- Document the doses and effects of the medications for future reference.
- Maintain a high index of suspicion for adverse effects of psychotropic medications.
- Review the rationale for ongoing prescription annually or more frequently.

Withdrawal from antipsychotic medication

In some cases, psychotropic medication (particularly benzodiazepines and antipsychotics) can be significantly reduced or even stopped. Withdrawal of psychotropic medication may need to be carried out gradually if the patient has been on it long term. Reasons for withdrawing psychotropic medication include:

➤ if re-evaluation of the original and current reasons for prescription of the medication suggests little or no rationale for continued prescription
➤ if there has been no benefit after a reasonable trial at reasonable doses
➤ when the adverse effects of medication outweigh the benefits.

To withdraw a long-term antipsychotic (one taken for six months or more) decrease the original dose by 10% every two to three weeks, or more slowly if behavioural disturbance occurs after initial dose reduction. Tapering can occur more quickly if an atypical antipsychotic is being substituted. Substitution with one of the atypical antipsychotics (which have less propensity to cause extrapyramidal effects) should be considered where extrapyramidal effects are a problem.

To withdraw a short-term antipsychotic (one taken for less than six months) decrease the dose at a faster rate, e.g. 20% to 25% of the original dose every three to seven days.

Withdrawal reactions

Difficulties in withdrawal from long-term antipsychotic therapy are more likely if the patient has been on high doses (>100 mg of chlorpromazine or equivalent), or has stereotypies, hyperactivity or autism. Withdrawal from antipsychotics may result in a number of reactions.

➤ **Behavioural deterioration** – due to symptom flare-up of underlying psychosis – occurs within days to weeks of withdrawal and requires reinstatement of antipsychotic treatment.
➤ **Rebound akathisia** (motor restlessness and pacing) can be confused with psychosis or anxiety.
➤ **Withdrawal dyskinesias and dystonias** are typically facial movements – especially lip puckering and tongue movements – and more rarely dystonias and choreoathetoid movements of the limbs that can last for several months. There is no clinically validated effective treatment, apart from raising the dose of the antipsychotic agent.
➤ **Anticholinergic withdrawal symptoms** include loss of appetite, nausea, vomiting, diarrhoea and agitation. These occur most often with thioridazine and chlorpromazine withdrawal.

Investigations prior to treatment with psychotropic medication

The choice of investigations to undertake prior to commencing treatment with psychotropic medications is a clinical judgement; it should take into account the past and current medical history, physical examination findings and the medication to be prescribed. Before prescribing antipsychotics, mood stabilisers or antidepressants, consider the following baseline investigations:

➤ urea and electrolytes
➤ full blood count
➤ liver function tests
➤ thyroid function tests
➤ blood lipids and glucose
➤ prolactin level
➤ weight and BP
➤ electrocardiogram (if there is a history of cardiac disorder).

Some people with intellectual disability may refuse blood tests; sometimes these investigations can only be done with sedation or under a general anaesthetic or lorazepam given orally 1–2 mg two hours before and another 1 mg given immediately before. If this is the case, medications such as lithium should not be prescribed unless there is no alternative.

Treatment in situations of diagnostic uncertainty

In situations of diagnostic uncertainty, patterns of behaviours (sometimes referred to as 'behavioural equivalents' of psychiatric symptoms) may suggest a psychiatric disorder is present. For example, a non-verbal person with repeated episodes of reduced sleep, increased vocalisation, increased masturbation and increased activity such as pacing, absconding or stripping, with a positive family history of bipolar disorder would suggest a presumptive diagnosis of mania provided medical causes were excluded. Psychiatric assessment is advised and a trial of standard antimanic therapy should be considered.

Psychotic disorders

Antipsychotic medications are indicated for psychotic disorders, mania and psychotic depression. Adverse effects are common, but there is a wide range of individual differences in their occurrence.

Amisulpride, aripiprazole, clozapine, olanzapine, quetiapine, risperidone and ziprasidone are referred to as atypical antipsychotics. Apart from clozapine, these antipsychotics appear to be at least as effective as the typical drugs in the treatment of psychoses, but are better tolerated, are less likely to cause extrapyramidal adverse effects and may be more efficacious for the negative symptoms and cognitive deficits of schizophrenia. Clozapine has superior efficacy compared to the typical antipsychotics but, because of its adverse effect profile, it should be reserved for use in treatment-resistant patients and those at increased risk of suicide.

It is important to note, however, that atypical antipsychotics have some significant limitations and complications; their benefits compared to both each other, and to the typical antipsychotics, are not always clear-cut. Adverse effects of antipsychotic medications may be either unrecognised or misdiagnosed in people with developmental disability. They all have adverse effects on lipid levels and glucose

TABLE 15.1 Relative frequency of common adverse effects of antipsychotics at usual therapeutic doses

Drug	Usual daily oral dose range (mg)	Anticholinergic	Dyslipidaemia	Extrapyramidal	Hyperglycaemia	Orthostatic hypotension	Sedation	Weight gain
Second-generation drugs								
amisulpride	400 to 1000 (acute psychosis) 100 to 300 (negative symptoms)	0	?	++ [NB1]	+	+	+	+
aripiprazole	15 to 30	0	0	+	0	+	+	+
clozapine	200 to 600	+++	+++	+	+++	++	+++	+++
olanzapine	5 to 30 [NB2]	+++	+++	+	+++	+	+++	+++
paliperidone	3 to 12	0	++	++	++	++ (initially)	++ (initially)	++
quetiapine	300 to 750	++	++	+ [NB1]	+++	++	+++	++
risperidone	2 to 6	0	++	++	++	++ (initially)	++ (initially)	++
ziprasidone	80 to 160	+	0	+	+	++	++	+
First-generation drugs								
chlorpromazine	75 to 500	+++	+++	++	+++	+++	+++	+++
droperidol	5 to 10 (IM) [NB3]	+	?	+++	?	+	++	+
haloperidol	1 to 7.5	+	+	+++	++	+	+	++
pericyazine	15 to 75	+++	?	+	+	++	+++	++
trifluoperazine	5 to 20	++	?	+++	+	++	+	++
zuclopenthixol acetate	50 to 150 (IM) [NB4]	++	?	++	+	+	+++	++
zuclopenthixol dihydrochloride	10 to 75	++	?	++	+	+	+++	++

Approximate frequencies of adverse effects: ? = no information or little reported; 0 (<2%) = negligible or absent; + (>2%) = infrequent; ++ (>10%) = moderately frequent; +++ (>30%) = frequent.

NB1: rarely a problem at usual therapeutic doses; NB2: maximum dose in accepted usage is greater than the maximum suggested in the manufacturer's product information; NB3: doses greater than 5 mg should not be given without immediate access to ECG monitoring and resuscitation facilities; NB4: single dose, not to be repeated for 2 to 3 days.

TABLE 15.2 Relative frequency of common adverse effects of depot antipsychotics at usual therapeutic doses

Drug	Usual IM dose range (mg) [NB1]	Dosing interval (weeks)	Anticholin-ergic	Dyslipidae-mia	Extrapy-ramidal	Hypergly-caemia	Orthostatic hypotension	Sedation	Weight gain
flupenthixol decanoate	20 to 40	2 to 4	++	?	+++	++	+	+	++
fluphenazine decanoate	12.5 to 50	2 to 4	+	?	+++	++	+	+	+++
haloperidol decanoate	50 to 200	4	+	+	+++	++	+	+	++
risperidone microspheres	25 to 50	2	0	++	++	++	+	+	++
zuclopenthixol decanoate	200 to 400 [NB2]	2 to 4	++	?	++	+	+	+++	++

Approximate frequencies of adverse effects: ? = no information or little reported; 0 (<2%) = negligible or absent; + (>2%) = infrequent; ++ (>10%) = moderately frequent; +++ (>30%) = frequent.

NB1: an initial test dose is recommended for all long-acting drugs (see #[Long-acting or depot antipsychotics in prevention of relapse]) especially if the patient has not been exposed to the class of antipsychotic drug previously.

NB2: patients switched from zuclopenthixol acetate do not require a test dose of zuclopenthixol decanoate.

Note: this is the frequency of occurrence of adverse effects, not the intensity with which they occur.

tolerance because they cause insulin resistance. Regular monitoring of weight, glucose levels, lipid levels and blood pressure are therefore essential aspects of regular healthcare and annual health checks.

Extrapyramidal effects

Extrapyramidal effects of antipsychotics include acute dystonias, akathisia, parkinsonism, tardive dyskinesia and neuroleptic (antipsychotic) malignant syndrome. Extrapyramidal adverse effects can increase the risk of falls and injury in people who already have impaired mobility and coordination.

The risk of antipsychotic-induced tardive dyskinesia is higher in people with organic brain syndromes and therefore probably more likely in people with developmental disability. Occasionally, abnormal movements similar to tardive dyskinesia may be present prior to treatment with antipsychotics, possibly due to cerebral pathology associated with the psychotic disorder.

In a person with intellectual disability, the early symptoms of the potentially fatal antipsychotic malignant syndrome may be missed.

There are some adverse effects of antipsychotics that may be confused for psychiatric symptoms, namely:

➤ akathisia – frequently not diagnosed, or misdiagnosed as anxiety or psychotic behaviour, and may result in increased prescription of antipsychotics, thus worsening the problem
➤ bradykinesia and immobile facies of parkinsonism – may be confused with symptoms of severe depression
➤ dysphoric (low) mood – frequently seen and may heighten pre-existing problems or mimic psychiatric disorders such as mood disturbance
➤ seizures – most antipsychotics reduce the seizure threshold. Some seizures (e.g. complex partial seizures) may present as increased behavioural disturbance and be interpreted as the psychiatric disorder worsening.

Mood disorders
Depressive disorders

Depressive disorders are frequently unrecognised in people with intellectual disability; consequently antidepressants are underprescribed. Depression should be assertively treated.

In people with moderate, severe or profound intellectual disability, antidepressants may lead to adverse reactions manifesting as behavioural disturbance, including transient generalised excitement and agitation, and an increase in frequency of aggressive, self-injurious or repetitive behaviours.

People with intellectual disability appear to be at some risk of having a hypomanic, manic or psychotic episode triggered by antidepressants. Care should be taken before prescribing antidepressants to exclude a past history suggestive of manic or hypomanic episodes or psychosis. If a bipolar disorder or psychosis is suspected, antidepressants may still be used with caution.

If manic symptoms emerge, the antidepressant dose should be reduced or ceased. If mania persists, treatment for a manic episode is indicated.

A psychiatric opinion is required when:

➤ the person has attempted suicide or has suicidal ideation
➤ psychotic symptoms are present

➤ the person is at risk from self-neglect and inadequate oral intake
➤ treatment triggers a manic episode
➤ the depression is treatment resistant.

There is little research-based evidence to support the use of one group of anti-depressants over another in people with intellectual disability and the choice of antidepressant remains a clinical judgement. Careful appraisal of the potential adverse effect profile of a particular antidepressant in conjunction with the present-ing symptoms, other medications and the general medical state of the patient help to guide choice of treatment.

SELECTIVE SEROTONIN REUPTAKE INHIBITORS

SSRIs are widely used in the treatment of depression in people with intellectual dis-ability; they are an acceptable first-line treatment. SSRIs may interact with a range of other medications, including other psychotropic medications. Citalopram has the least potential for drug–drug interactions, followed by sertraline.

Agitated or aggressive behaviour may occasionally worsen with an SSRI; as SSRIs do not usually cause sedation; mirtazapine may be preferred when night-time sedation is needed. SSRIs may also cause nausea, loss of appetite and weight loss.

To minimise adverse effects, start on a very low dose and gradually increase. Citalopram can be started at 10 mg (sertraline at 25 mg) per day to allow flexibility of dosing.

There are no studies regarding the use of mirtazapine, mianserin, venlafaxine or reboxetine in people with intellectual disability. However, these medications have been used safely in the elderly and are therefore acceptable choices for the treatment of depression in people with intellectual disability.

TRICYCLIC ANTIDEPRESSANTS

When used to treat major depression, tricyclic antidepressants (TCAs) can be very effective treatments, although there are a number of adverse effects that may be particularly problematic in people with intellectual disability. Adverse effects that may cause particular problems are:
➤ impaired cognition
➤ hypotension and blurred vision – which may lead to falls
➤ difficulty with micturition, incontinence or urinary retention
➤ constipation
➤ weight gain
➤ sedation
➤ lowered seizure threshold – leading to cognitive difficulties
➤ irritability and aggression.

These adverse effects may all result in challenging behaviour.

MONOAMINE OXIDASE INHIBITORS

There are no studies available on the efficacy and safety of the irreversible mono-amine oxidase inhibitors (MAOIs) phenelzine and tranylcypromine in people with intellectual disability. The dietary restrictions required when using irreversible MAOIs limit their potential usefulness in people who do not have the ability or reliable support to monitor diet as needed. They should not be prescribed without psychiatric consultation.

The reversible MAOI, moclobemide, has been used successfully in the elderly without impairing cognitive function. However, there are no studies available on the efficacy and safety of moclobemide in people with intellectual disability.

ELECTROCONVULSIVE THERAPY

Intellectual disability per se is not a contraindication to electroconvulsive therapy. There are no controlled trials; however, case reports indicate that electroconvulsive therapy is both effective and safe for mood disorders in people with intellectual disability and, in particular, for depression with psychotic symptoms.

Bipolar disorder

Acute mania and hypomania both appear to be more common in people with intellectual disability and are often misdiagnosed as schizophrenia or as 'behavioural' disturbance. Antipsychotics are used in conjunction with mood stabilisers such as lithium and antiepileptics. Benzodiazepines may also be used in the early stages of treatment of acute manic episodes. Mood stabilisers have prophylactic effects that are not found with the antipsychotics.

Bipolar disorders are not infrequently misdiagnosed as schizophrenia or as 'behavioural' disturbance in people with intellectual disability.

Where there is a bipolar or cycling pattern of disturbed behaviour, mood stabilisers – rather than antipsychotics – are the treatment of choice for long-term management. Antipsychotics should be reduced to the lowest effective dosage and withdrawn if possible.

MOOD STABILISERS

Currently lithium, sodium valproate and carbamazepine are used as mood stabilisers in the treatment of acute mania and the prophylaxis of bipolar disorder. They can be used in people with intellectual disability.

If the serum levels and adverse effects can be monitored regularly and reliably, lithium is the drug of first choice for mood stabilisation. Sodium valproate is most effective for rapid cycling bipolar disorders (i.e. four or more episodes of mood disturbance in a 12-month period).

In patients with epilepsy who are already on sodium valproate or carbamazepine, and who develop a bipolar disorder, it would be prudent to attempt mood stabilisation by increasing the dose of the antiepileptic.

LITHIUM

Lithium has a number of disadvantages relative to the other mood stabilisers including the need for regular serum level monitoring, risk of central nervous system toxicity and hypothyroidism (which may be missed more easily in someone with intellectual disability). The care arrangements, stability and training of staff need to be carefully assessed before prescribing lithium.

It is, however, used as a mood stabiliser with good therapeutic effect in many patients with intellectual disability who have bipolar disorder.

Lithium requires regular serum level monitoring; serum lithium levels should fall within the lower range 0.4 to 0.8 mmol/L, except in acute episodes of mania when higher levels of 0.8 to 1 mmol/L should be aimed for. Thyroid and renal function monitoring should also be done regularly.

Inform carers of the importance of:
➤ regular monitoring of serum lithium levels
➤ checking or stopping the drug if the patient becomes febrile, sweats heavily or loses fluids (e.g. severe vomiting or diarrhoea)
➤ the potential for adverse drug interactions (e.g. with diuretics and nonsteroidal anti-inflammatory drugs).

Acute lithium toxicity is more likely with serum levels over 1.3 mmol/L, but toxicity can also occur at therapeutic levels. Toxicity symptoms include coarse tremor, ataxia, dysarthria, confusion, muscle weakness, diarrhoea, vomiting, renal impairment and cardiac arrhythmias.

SODIUM VALPROATE AND CARBAMAZEPINE

Although there is no clear evidence for the most effective serum concentrations of these mood stabilisers in bipolar disorder, concentrations of 50 to 100 mg/L (350 to 700 micromol/L) for sodium valproate and 4 to 12 mg/L (17 to 50 micromol/L) for carbamazepine are used as guidelines.

Baseline haematology, renal and liver function should be assessed prior to commencing these medications. It is good practice to monitor serum levels, blood count and liver function every six months.

Adverse effects of sodium valproate include nausea, diarrhoea, change in appetite, headache, sedation, blurred vision, tremor, ataxia, hair loss, menstrual irregularities, hepatotoxicity and impaired clotting.

Carbamazepine's adverse effects include an increase in behavioural problems, worsening of seizures, rash, sedation, ataxia, gastrointestinal upset, hepatic dysfunction and, rarely, neutropenia.

COMBINATIONS OF MOOD STABILISERS

If monotherapy with one of the standard mood stabilisers is ineffective, combination therapy may be indicated. Expert psychiatric assessment is recommended.

Anxiety disorders

Anxiety is frequently present in individuals with intellectual disability; it can occur as a symptom or as a psychiatric disorder. High levels of anxiety may result in agitation, increased repetitive behaviours or even aggression. Excess anxiety is often associated with autism spectrum disorders. Organic and medical factors (e.g. caffeinism, hyperthyroidism) must be excluded. Anxiety can be managed by pharmacological and non-pharmacological methods, or a combination of both.

Obsessive-compulsive disorder, generalised anxiety disorder, phobic disorders, panic disorder and post-traumatic stress disorder all occur in people with intellectual disability.

Non-pharmacological management

Non-pharmacological methods are important to consider. They may be more helpful than pharmacological treatments in the long term. Approaches include:
➤ the use of cognitive and behavioural therapies

➤ training in anxiety management and relaxation techniques
➤ environmental manipulations (e.g. preparation of the individual for changes in routine)
➤ educating support persons to handle anxiety-provoking situations more effectively
➤ the use of breathing control techniques at times of panic episodes or comorbid panic disorder.

Carers are often not aware of the anxiety and fear that someone with intellectual disability may have. It may be possible to discover anxiety symptoms (including physiological signs) by careful mental state and physical examinations.

Pharmacological agents may help with non-pharmacological interventions.

Pharmacological management

There are currently no ideal pharmacological treatments for long-term management of generalised anxiety in people with intellectual disability. Benzodiazepines, the most commonly prescribed treatments, are associated with the adverse effects of withdrawal symptoms after long-term use. Where anxiety occurs with depression, an SSRI may produce anxiolytic, as well as antidepressant, actions without the problems of dependence.

Three pharmacological approaches to the management of generalised anxiety are discussed below.

BENZODIAZEPINES

Benzodiazepines are widely prescribed and may have good short-term effect in acute anxiety. Unfortunately, a small proportion of people with intellectual disability become paradoxically aroused, agitated and disinhibited on benzodiazepines; these medications should be avoided in such sensitive individuals.

Benzodiazepines also cause sedation, impaired cognition, dizziness, psychomotor retardation, weakness, unsteadiness and disorientation; these adverse effects are particularly troublesome to those with impaired cognitive function. Benzodiazepines also cause dependence when prescribed long term, and the withdrawal state can be extended and extremely distressing for the patient. They should only be prescribed for very limited periods for the short-term management of acute situations.

BUSPIRONE

Buspirone is an anxiolytic that may be useful when treatment is long term. The cost of prescription needs to be considered. Buspirone does not cause dependence. It cannot be used to cover benzodiazepine withdrawal. Buspirone takes two to four weeks to take effect:
➤ 5 mg orally, three times a day initially, increasing if necessary to 20 mg three times a day and continuing for several weeks after symptoms subside so the patient can adjust to a life with lower anxiety. The mean effective daily dose of buspirone is 20 to 25 mg.

The most common adverse effects include drowsiness, dizziness, light-headedness, nausea and headache. It is not possible to predict which patients will respond to buspirone and it should be considered a second-line treatment.

PROPRANOLOL

Propranolol, a beta-blocker, 10 to 40 mg orally, three times daily, can reduce the somatic effects of anxiety such as palpitations and sweating. It may be useful in individuals who experience significant somatic symptoms of anxiety:

Adverse effects include exacerbation of asthma, hypotension and worsening of cardiac failure and propranolol should not be used when these conditions are present.

Hyperprolactinaemia as a side-effect of psychotropic medication

Hyperprolactinaemia can be due to stress including the stress of phlebotomy, other associated endocrine disorders, pituitary tumours or drugs. It can result in hypogonadism resulting especially in an increased risk of osteoporosis/osteopenia already more prevalent in adults with intellectual disability.

➤ *Severe* – 2000 or more results in hypogonadism, galactorrhoea, amenorrhoea
➤ *Moderate* – 1000–2000 results in oligoamenorrhoea.

BOX 15.2 Causes of hyperprolactinaemia

- Stress
- Functioning pituitary adenoma:
  - microadenoma*
  - macroadenoma
- Hypothyroidism
- Polycystic ovary disease
- Non-functioning pituitary adenoma – stalk effect
- Pregnancy
- Intercourse
- CKD 4/5
- Liver disease
- Trauma to nipple or chest wall nearby
- Drugs

BOX 15.3 Consequences of hyperprolactinaemia

- Osteopenia/osteoporosis
- Weight gain
- Amenorrhoea
- Gynaecomastia
- Galactorrhoea
- Loss of hair and muscle mass and oligospermia in men

TABLE 15.3 Drugs which cause hyperprolactinaemia

Psychotropic agents	Others – moderate increases only
	Opiates
NEUROLEPTICS – high levels	Verapamil
Thioridazine	Methyl dopa
Chlorpromazine	Protease inhibitor antivirals
Haloperidol	Bezafibrate
Sulpiride	Omeprazole
Amisulpride	H2 Antagonists
Fluphenazine	Dopamine receptor blockers:
Flupenthixol	– metoclopramide
Risperidone	– domperidone
ANTIDEPRESSANTS – variable effect	
Tricyclics	
SS SSRIs	
MAOIs	

Stopping a drug for three days will usually be associated with a fall in prolactin level but this can be a difficult decision to make when the patient has been treated with a neuroleptic, so consideration should be given to using drugs which do not result in hyperprolactinaemia, especially in women who are particularly at risk of osteoporosis.

BOX 15.4 Neuroleptic drugs which do not usually cause increase in prolactin

- Clozapine
- Quetiapine
- Olanzapine
- Aripiprazole
- Ziprasidone

It is useful to differentiate between hyperprolactinaemia due to drugs and that due to a macroprolactinoma – a large invasive pituitary tumour. Microadenomas are not associated with any space-occupying features.

BOX 15.5 Consequences of macroprolactinoma

- Headaches
- Visual field defect progressing to blindness
- Stalk effect resulting in loss of inhibition of prolactin
- Hypopituitarism
- Cranial nerve palsies
- CSF leaks and secondary meningitis

So ideally a prolactin level should be done:
➤ as a baseline
➤ three months after starting an at risk drug
➤ three months after the dose of an at risk drug is increased
➤ three days and three weeks after an at risk drug is stopped or reduced in dosage
➤ to any patient with suggestive symptoms at any time.

But the specimens need to be taken when the patient is not stressed by the phlebotomy.

If an elevated prolactin level is obtained from a patient treated with a neuroleptic agent each patient has to be managed individually but the following management plan could be used.

Repeat level under calmest circumstances possible.
At same time do thyroid function tests and FSH/LH as screen for PCOS and ask for macroprolactin level.

Level still elevated and no evidence of thyroid disease or PCOS.
Macroprolactin level grossly elevated. No further action needed – monitor prolactin as before, assuming normal level.

(Macroprolactin is a large molecule form of prolactin which has much less effect and it has nothing specifically to do with macroprolactinomas.)

Level still elevated and no evidence of thyroid disease or PCOS.
Macroprolactin not elevated.
Consider risk based on repeated levels (levels in mIU/L):
➤ <530 normal in women <424 normal in men
➤ antipsychotics can cause level of 3000 and even up to 6000
➤ >3000 tumour likely
➤ 3000–6000 with an MRI scan showing a macroadenoma is due to an adenoma producing prolactin or an adenoma damaging the pituitary stalk thereby reducing the effect of prolactin inhibiting hormone. Treatment of the tumour by drugs, radiotherapy or surgery needs to be considered
➤ drug induced – usually less than 5000
➤ >6000 diagnostic of tumour.

Consider presence of symptoms suggesting presence of macroadenoma. In the presence of these but only a moderately elevated prolactin level remember the 'hook effect' (j curve effect) – massively elevated levels of prolactin are recorded on the assays as only moderately elevated levels.

If the prolactin level is still elevated discussions between all involved in the care of the patient need to consider performing a perimetry to pick up a pituitary tumour, doing an MRI scan to fine a macroadenoma, changing the neuroleptic and following the prolactin level or even accepting the hyperprolactinaemia and protecting the patient against osteoporosis with bisphosphonates.

FURTHER READING

- Aziz M, Maixner DF, DeQuardo J, *et al.* ECT and mental retardation: a review and case reports. *J ECT.* 2001; **17**(2): 149–52.
- Crabbe HC. Pharmacotherapy in mental retardation. In: Bouras N, editor. *Mental Health in Mental Retardation: recent advances and practices.* Cambridge: Cambridge University Press; 1994.
- Cutajar P, Wilson D. The use of ECT in intellectual disability. *J Intellect Disabil Res.* 1999; **43**(5): 421–7.
- Einfeld SL. Clinical assessment of psychiatric symptoms in mentally retarded individuals. *Aust N Z J Psychiatry.* 1992; **26**(1): 48–63.
- Holt RIG. Medical causes and consequences of hyperprolactinaemia. A context for psychiatrists. *J Psychopharmacol.* 2008; **22**(Suppl. 2): S28–37.
- Peveler RC. Antipsychotics and hyperprolactinaemia: clinical recommendations. *J Psychopharmacol.* **22**(Suppl. 2): S98–103 and other contributions to supplement; 2008.
- Serri O, Chik CL, Ur E, *et al.* Diagnosis and management of hyperprolactinaemia. *Can Med Assoc J.* 2003; **16**: 169.

CHAPTER 16

Epilepsy

Epilepsy occurs at a much higher than normal frequency in people with intellectual disability; it is often more severe and more difficult to control than it is in other people. Between 25% and 35% of people with intellectual disability also have epilepsy, compared to approximately 2% of the general population.

Although the combination of intellectual disability and epilepsy makes the diagnosis and management of epilepsy a challenging area, it is usually possible to achieve satisfactory control of seizures without excessive adverse effects by using one antiepileptic drug at a time. The choice of this drug needs to be based on an accurate classification of the seizure type and attention needs to be paid to subtle signs of adverse effects. This chapter describes issues of management and treatment pertinent to people with intellectual disability.

Although most people with epilepsy need some degree of specialist overview of their management, the GP is well placed to play a major role in coordinating diagnosis and treatment.

EPILEPSY AND SPECIFIC SYNDROMES

Although many people with intellectual disability and epilepsy have an unknown aetiology for their conditions, there are several identifiable syndromes in which epilepsy is more common:

➤ Tuberous sclerosis is characterised by a triad of features – skin manifestations, intellectual disability and epilepsy. It is a multisystem genetic disease in which there are tuber-like growths in the brain and other major organs.

➤ Down syndrome has a bimodal onset – in 40% of people, seizures occur before one year of age, and in another 40% they occur in the third decade of life.

➤ Fragile X syndrome is the most commonly known inherited cause of intellectual disability and results in a wide variety of presentations. Fragile X syndrome is confirmed by DNA testing.

➤ Lennox-Gastaut syndrome is characterised by multiple seizure types (atypical absence, tonic, atonic) and generalised slow spike-and-wave discharges on EEG; it can be due to a number of causes. For management recommendations, *see* p. 143.

➤ Angelman syndrome is a neurodevelopmental disorder characterised by a peculiar ataxic gait and puppet-like movements, and is associated with severe intellectual disability, microcephaly, speech impairments and seizures. Angelman syndrome is confirmed by DNA testing.

Epilepsy is also more common in cerebral palsy – a persistent (but not unchanging) disorder of movement and posture due to a defect or lesion of the developing brain. Cerebral palsy may be associated with coexisting intellectual disability.

Further information may also be seen in individual chapters on syndromes and cerebral palsy.

DIAGNOSIS

The diagnosis of epilepsy is by clinical means, with augmentation by special investigations. The mainstay of rational prescribing of antiepileptic drugs is accurate diagnosis with proper categorisation of seizure type and (where possible) the specific epilepsy syndrome. This may be particularly difficult in people with intellectual disability due to:

➤ communication problems that hinder obtaining an accurate history
➤ fragmentation and unreliability of information that may be provided
➤ behavioural issues that cloud the clinical picture
➤ poor tolerance of investigative procedures by the patient.

History taking

If there are barriers to communication, it is important to gather information from several sources, and defer decisions about diagnosis and treatment until the person who knows the patient best (often a parent or key worker) has been interviewed. The history should include:

➤ a description of seizures, including their frequency and duration
➤ any relevant environmental circumstances
➤ antecedents to, and patterns of, the seizures (e.g. premenstrual exacerbation of seizures)
➤ whether the seizures are getting worse, better or staying the same
➤ whether the seizures have been constant, or if they have remitted and recurred over time.

Differential diagnosis

In some situations, it will be unclear whether a person's actions (episodic behaviour disturbance, falls, prolonged staring or periodic unresponsiveness) are due to epilepsy, or to other factors including problem behaviours, psychiatric disorders, muscle spasms, paroxysmal movement disorders, syncope, sleep disorders and migraine. Problem behaviours are often the most difficult to exclude as a cause of the person's action; nevertheless, specific factors in the history may help in differentiating between epileptic seizures and pseudoseizures that occur as a result of behavioural outbursts (*see* Table 16.1).

TABLE 16.1 Differentiating factors of behavioural pseudoseizures and epileptic seizures

Differentiating factors	Pseudoseizures	Seizures
Antecedents	Often (but not always) there are clear external triggers such as interpersonal conflicts, change in routine or environment	Sleep deprivation, fever, alcohol, photic stimulation, missed medication Often no obvious or apparent trigger
Characteristics	May be bizarre or stylised movements	Specific seizure type is usually recognisable
Conscious state	May respond to certain stimuli	Usually unconscious
Incontinence	Unusual	Common
Injury during seizure	Unusual	Common
Recovery	Rapid and complete	Often postictal confusion
Setting	May occur more often in one setting than another, or in the presence of certain people only	Occur equally in all settings

In situations when the history fails to clarify the diagnosis, combined EEG and video monitoring may be helpful.

Investigations
Electroencephalogram
While not an invasive procedure, obtaining an EEG – even without video monitoring – is a restrictive process that may be frightening to a person with intellectual disability, and difficult to accomplish in a person with cerebral palsy or autism. Desensitisation (involving repeated visits to the EEG suite and gradual introduction to the technician and equipment) is time-consuming but may be beneficial. Oral sedation may be necessary; the choice of drug is best discussed with the EEG technician. EEG under general anaesthetic is rarely useful because of interference from anaesthetic drugs.

In the presence of strong clinical evidence, inability to obtain an EEG, or obtaining an EEG that does not show classical epileptiform activity, should not prevent a diagnosis of epilepsy.

Neuroimaging
Structural neuroimaging using computerised tomography (CT) and magnetic resonance imaging (MRI) has a critical role in determining the aetiology and location of origin of seizures. Patients may require sedation or anaesthesia. MRI is particularly useful in detecting abnormalities of cortical development, which are frequent causes of epilepsy and developmental disability. Some clinicians use MRI in all cases of idiopathic intellectual disability, as a demonstration of structural lesions potentially assists in making a definitive diagnosis of the underlying syndrome, as well as assisting in the management of the epilepsy.

Single photon emission computed tomography (SPECT) and positron emission tomography (PET) have no routine role in evaluation.

CLASSIFICATION OF SEIZURES

When treating epilepsy it is important to accurately diagnose the seizure type (*see* Table 16.2) and when possible the epilepsy syndrome (*see* Table 16.3) using EEG and appropriate neuroimaging, as seizure type determines the antiepileptic drug of choice (*see* Table 16.4).

TABLE 16.2 Classification of epileptic seizures

Generalised seizures	Partial seizures
Absence	Simple partial
Myoclonic	Complex partial
Tonic-clonic	Secondarily generalised
Tonic	
Atonic	

Based on the International League Against Epilepsy classification of epileptic seizures.

TABLE 16.3 Classification of epileptic syndromes

Generalised epilepsies
Symptomatic generalised
West syndrome (infantile spasms, hypsarrhythmia)
Lennox-Gastaut syndrome

Primary generalised
Childhood absence epilepsy
Juvenile absence epilepsy
Juvenile myoclonic epilepsy
Epilepsy with tonic-clonic seizures on awakening

Partial epilepsies
Symptomatic (e.g. mesial temporal lobe epilepsy)
Idiopathic (e.g. benign childhood epilepsy with centrotemporal spikes)

Epilepsies undetermined whether partial or generalised
Neonatal seizures
Tonic-clonic seizures (clinical and EEG findings do not permit classification as generalised or partial onset)

Special syndromes
Febrile seizures
Isolated seizure or status epilepticus
Metabolic seizures and toxic-induced seizures

Based on the International League Against Epilepsy classification of epileptic syndromes.

People with intellectual disability may have any seizure type; many experience more than one type.

MANAGEMENT

Seizures may be particularly resistant to treatment in people with intellectual disability, but there is no link between the severity of a person's intellectual disability and the severity of their seizure disorder.

Antiepileptic drug treatment

Treatment of epilepsy with antiepileptic drugs may be more difficult in people with intellectual disability than in the general population; the difficulty of discriminating seizures from other phenomena may complicate the use of antiepileptic drugs.

Most clinicians recommend antiepileptic drug treatment for people who have experienced two or more seizures. This decision may be different for people with intellectual disability for a number of reasons:

➤ Most people with intellectual disability do not drive cars or operate heavy machinery, and many are supervised in potentially dangerous situations, resulting in a lesser risk of traumatic consequences of a seizure.

➤ People with intellectual disability are at a greater risk of adverse effects from antiepileptic drugs.

➤ While there is evidence that epileptic seizures are rarely dangerous in people without intellectual disability, mortality is increased in people who have both intellectual disability and epilepsy due to a concurrent increase in comorbidities (such as heart or lung disease).

➤ People with more severe disabilities (such as spastic quadriplegia) and epilepsy are at significantly increased risk of death if their seizures are poorly controlled.

➤ The phenomenon of sudden unexpected death in epilepsy is still poorly understood but it occurs often enough to warrant extreme diligence in the control of seizures.

➤ Structural cerebral lesions are associated with a greater risk of recurrent seizures (epilepsy).

The decision to treat a person needs to be based on a careful analysis of the likely impact of seizures on a person's health and quality of life, and the likelihood and impact of adverse effects of antiepileptic drugs.

A summary of the common epileptic seizure types and the antiepileptic drugs of first choice is shown in Table 16.4.

TABLE 16.4 Common epileptic seizure types and antiepileptic drugs of first choice

Seizure type	Antiepileptic drug
Absence	Ethosuximide (absence only)
	Sodium valproate (absence and tonic-clonic)
Myoclonic	Sodium valproate
Tonic-clonic:	
generalised	Sodium valproate
secondarily generalised	Carbamazepine
undetermined if generalised or partial	Carbamazepine, sodium valproate
Simple partial	Carbamazepine
Complex partial	Carbamazepine

Drug choice

The following factors must be considered when choosing an antiepileptic drug for a person with intellectual disability.

➤ **Efficacy**: Choosing the drug most likely to be efficacious requires careful determination of seizure type and epilepsy syndrome. There may be multiple or complex types of seizures present.

➤ **Adverse effect profile**: The intellectually disabled population is particularly sensitive to neurological adverse effects, but may have difficulty communicating the adverse effects.

➤ **Probability of interactions**: Many people with intellectual disability are on more than one medication.

➤ **Ease of use**: Consider the form of the drug, route of administration, frequency of dosing and need for plasma level monitoring. Intolerance of blood tests and poor compliance with antiepileptic drugs complicate their use, as does the involvement of support persons who are inadequately trained and unable to recognise subtle seizures.

➤ **Expense**: Treatment is usually long term and cost may be an issue.

Rational use of antiepileptic drugs

Most people with intellectual disability can have their epilepsy controlled by one – or at most two – antiepileptic drugs. If combination therapy is required, a second antiepileptic drug should be chosen to complement the first drug; attention should be paid to each drug's influence on the other's metabolism. Monotherapy with the most appropriate antiepileptic drug should be pursued as far as possible before changing to, or adding, other agents.

Care should be taken to find the minimum effective dose for antiepileptic drugs, and to cease drugs which are clearly non-efficacious. Reduction of antiepileptics in those with intellectual disability and epilepsy who are receiving a complex drug regimen has been associated with better seizure control and, anecdotally, improved behaviour and social interaction.

A routine clinical review should be scheduled every three months for people using an antiepileptic drug. All antiepileptics can occasionally and paradoxically increase seizure frequency.

Table 16.4 shows the antiepileptic drug of first choice according to seizure type.

Adverse effects of antiepileptic drugs

Adverse effects commonly result from the use of antiepileptic drugs, especially in people with intellectual disability. Monitor for adverse effects clinically rather than biochemically.

A careful history and examination is more reliable than measuring plasma levels of most antiepileptic drugs. The plasma levels of most drugs usually contribute little to management, and they should be requested and interpreted in this light. The exception is phenytoin, which has non-linear pharmacokinetics; it can reach toxic levels with small increases in dose.

Adverse effects that might indicate the need for dose reduction are ataxia, dysarthria, drowsiness, decline in cognition, agitation and other disturbed behaviours.

Some adverse effects are of particular relevance to people with intellectual disability.

➤ Gingival hypertrophy, which occurs in approximately 30% of people who use phenytoin. As people with intellectual disability often have poor oral health anyway, vigilance is required.

➤ Aggression may be stimulated in people with intellectual disability by both vigabatrin and clonazepam.
➤ Severe skin diseases (including Stevens-Johnson syndrome) can occasionally be caused by lamotrigine.
➤ Severe weight loss can be caused by topiramate.

ANTIEPILEPTICS AND COGNITION

In addition to the cognitive effects of the underlying condition, the effects of other medications and the effects of poor seizure control, antiepileptics can alter cognition in their own right. The impact on the person with intellectual disability can be severe.

Adverse cognitive effects of antiepileptic drugs are associated with polypharmacy, and also with the use of phenobarbitone – some doctors choose to avoid phenobarbitone because of its very high incidence of cognitive impairment. Phenytoin, sodium valproate and carbamazepine are associated with a similar degree of generally mild psychomotor slowing.

The cognitive effects of the newer antiepileptic drugs in people with intellectual disability are less clear; they cannot necessarily be assumed from studies in those without cognitive impairment. In people without intellectual disability, topiramate has been demonstrated to adversely impact cognitive function, whereas lamotrigine (at least in the short term) appears to have few adverse effects and may activate cognition. The effects of the remaining newer antiepileptic drugs on cognition are uncertain.

Withdrawal of antiepileptic drugs

The withdrawal of antiepileptic drugs is a controversial area. Most people with epilepsy report significantly improved quality of life when, using antiepileptic drugs, their seizures are controlled, and many prefer to keep taking antiepileptic drugs indefinitely. People with intellectual disability who have well-controlled seizures and who do not experience significant adverse effects from their antiepileptic drugs may also be reluctant to cease them.

Both good seizure control through the use of monotherapy, and also stabilisation on the minimum effective dose of antiepileptic drugs, contribute to an improved quality of life.

If a person has been seizure-free for two to three years and is on a constant level of antiepileptic drugs, a very slow process of withdrawal may be undertaken. The process is more likely to be successful if the EEG is normal (although success varies even with a normal EEG), but the decision to withdraw medication should be based on clinical judgement rather than the absence of EEG abnormalities.

As people with intellectual disability usually have some brain pathology underlying their epilepsy, withdrawal of antiepileptic drugs is often less successful than in the rest of the population. Those with a structural cerebral lesion are less likely to remain seizure-free after ceasing antiepileptics. Also, because of difficulties in obtaining an accurate history, it is more difficult to be sure that seizures really are controlled.

Specific areas of management
LENNOX-GASTAUT SYNDROME

Lennox-Gastaut syndrome is characterised by the early onset and coexistence of many different forms of seizures that usually become progressively more difficult to control. The intellectual disability associated with it is usually severe.

The initial therapy of choice is:
➤ sodium valproate 30 mg/kg/day orally, in two divided doses, gradually increasing to 60 mg/kg/day, until seizures cease or adverse effects occur.

Lamotrigine (in lower than usual doses) or clonazepam may need to be added when seizures become more difficult to control.

Lamotrigine can be a very effective antiepileptic drug in Lennox-Gastaut syndrome, and its use should be considered in all cases. Use:
➤ lamotrigine
➤ adult: 25 mg orally, daily for two weeks, increase by 25 mg every two to four weeks up to 400 mg/day in two divided doses, until seizures cease or adverse effects occur.

Much lower doses of lamotrigine are needed if it is added to sodium valproate:
➤ lamotrigine (when added to sodium valproate)
➤ adult: 25 mg orally, on alternate days, for two weeks, increase by 25 mg every two to four weeks up to 200 mg/day in two divided doses, until seizures cease or adverse effects occur.

Higher lamotrigine doses may be required in some individuals.

Slow introduction minimises the risk of skin rash and allows support persons to determine the effects of each dose on alertness and seizure frequency.

If lamotrigine fails or cannot be tolerated, use:
➤ clonazepam
➤ adult: 1 mg orally, daily in divided doses, increase as necessary up to 6 mg, daily in divided doses

or
➤ topiramate
➤ adult: 25 mg orally, daily, for one week, increase by 25 mg each week, up to 200 mg daily.

Recent improvements in antiepileptic drugs make it important that all patients with Lennox-Gastaut syndrome are regularly reviewed by a neurologist who has expertise in epilepsy.

Status epilepticus
Status epilepticus refers to the situation in which a patient suffers from two or more generalised epileptic seizures without regaining consciousness between the seizures, or suffers from continuous partial seizures without clear cessation of epileptic activity between the seizures. It is a medical emergency.

Terminating status epilepticus requires the administration of:
➤ diazepam 10 to 20 mg bolus IV, not exceeding 2 to 5 mg/minute; repeat once 15 minutes later if status epilepticus continues

or
➤ clonazepam 1 to 2 mg bolus IV, not exceeding 0.5 mg/minute; repeat once 15 minutes later if status epilepticus continues

or
➤ midazolam 5 to 10 mg IM, repeat once 15 minutes later if status epilepticus continues

followed by
➤ phenytoin 15 to 20 mg/kg IV, not exceeding 50 mg/minute.

In cases where intravenous access is impossible, rectal diazepam may be given. Rectal diazepam can occasionally be a useful and safe treatment in patients with recurrent refractory tonic-clonic seizures. Family members or professional support persons may administer diazepam rectally, but they must be trained in its administration and do it according to clear guidelines.

Catamenial epilepsy

Some women may experience a premenstrual exacerbation of their seizure disorder due to fluctuations in endogenous hormones, or to a premenstrual fall in plasma antiepileptic drug concentration.

Antiepileptic drug-induced liver enzymes may affect the required amount of both the antiepileptic drugs and the drugs used to manage menstruation.

RECOMMENDATION

Chart seizures and menstrual cycles on a 12-month calendar to determine if there is an association, and consider increasing antiepileptic drug doses for the week prior to menstruation. On rare occasions, pharmacological regulation – or even suppression of menstruation – might be necessary to prevent premenstrual exacerbations of epilepsy.

Other management issues

Lifestyle

Seizures can be precipitated by sleep deprivation, flashing lights (e.g. disco, computer screens, television, bright sunlight), fever, dehydration, alcohol in excess, and illicit drugs. Optimal seizure control requires minimisation of precipitants, without imposing excessive restrictions that unnecessarily reduce the person's quality of life (e.g. people with epilepsy can go to discos or watch television with reasonable safety if sleep deprivation and excessive alcohol are avoided).

Safety

Uncontrolled seizures (especially if generalised) can be associated with trauma, or ill health as a consequence of fitting. People with epilepsy who have poor seizure control should not be allowed to swim or bathe unsupervised. Likewise, exposure to naked flames, cycling and adventure sports needs to be supervised or avoided.

FURTHER READING

• Aldenkamp AP, De Krom M, Reijs R. Newer antiepileptic drugs and cognitive issues. *Epilepsia*. 2003; **44**(Suppl. 4): 21–9.

CHAPTER 17

Nutritional disorders

Nutritional problems are common in people with intellectual disability, with both underweight and overweight occurring more frequently than in the general community. Underweight is commonly associated with dysphagia and more severe levels of physical limitations (e.g. in people with spastic quadriparesis); overweight and obesity, by contrast, are usually seen in people who have greater levels of mobility and functional independence. As in the general population, both underweight and overweight are associated with significant health consequences, and should not be accepted as being inherent to the disability.

People with intellectual disability are also at increased risk of specific vitamin and mineral deficiencies (such as deficiencies of vitamin D, iron and vitamin B_{12}).

There are no dietary guidelines that are specific to people with intellectual disability; the general population guidelines can be used as an initial reference point.

People with intellectual disability often have altered energy requirements that need consideration when making recommendations about dietary intake.

Nutritional disorders in people with intellectual disability can be complex, and their successful management requires a multidisciplinary approach that also includes the close involvement of family members and other support persons. The GP has an important role in the medical assessment and management, but may need to engage other clinicians such as gastroenterologists, speech pathologists and dieticians to ensure comprehensive assessment and management.

ASSESSMENT OF WEIGHT STATUS

Although anthropometry (height, weight, skin fold thickness and other body measurements) is an important component of nutritional assessment, it is insufficient on its own and needs to be considered with other information such as dietary intake, biochemical measures and the results of a clinical assessment.

NICE provides a weight for height chart that is useful in assessing the weight status of adults. People need to be able to stand upright without shoes for accurate height measurement.

Another measure that is commonly used to classify weight is body mass index (BMI):

$$BMI \ (kg/m^2) = Weight \ (kg)/height \ (m)^2$$

The World Health Organization (WHO) classification of BMI (for people of European descent) is outlined in Table 17.1. The BMI categories do not take into account differences in body build. The BMI range from 18.5 to 20 is more representative of people with a high activity level and good muscle tone (such as athletes) and those of particular ethnic origins (e.g. Asian).

For overweight and obese individuals with BMI<35, waist circumference is also a valid measure of disease risk; *see* Table 17.2.

TABLE 17.1 Classification of weight by body mass index (BMI)

Classification*	Body mass index (kg/m$_2$)	Risk of comorbidities
very underweight[†]	<17	very likely to have associated clinical problems
underweight	17–18.5	low (but possibly increased risk of other clinical problems)
normal range	18.5–24.9	average
overweight	>25	
– pre-obese	25–29.9	mildly increased
obese	≥30	
– grade I	30–34.9	moderate
– grade II	35–39.9	severe
– grade III	≥40	very severe

* Based on: World Health Organization. *Obesity: preventing and managing the global epidemic. Report of a WHO consultation.* WHO Technical Report Series Number 894. Geneva: WHO; 2000.

† This category is not in the WHO classification, but is used by Nutrition Australia in their Aim for the Healthy Weight Range chart.

TABLE 17.2 Waist circumference* at which risk increases

	Increased	Substantial increase
men	94 cm (OR 2.2)	102 cm (OR 4.6)
women	80 cm (OR 1.6)	88 cm (OR 2.6)

OR = odds ratio for increased risk of diseases associated with obesity.

* The figures given are for a population of European origin.

UNDERWEIGHT

Underweight is the manifestation of short-term or long-term undernutrition. As in the general population, short-term weight loss can occur during the course of an acute illness, or due to long-term serious disease resulting in cachexia. In a person with intellectual disability, chronic long-term underweight may be mistakenly ascribed to the disability, and thus accepted as part of the condition. Even though it is common for a person with severe disability to be underweight, it is not 'normal' and warrants intervention. Weight loss needs to be taken seriously and assessed fully, as for any other individual. The most common reason for persistent poor food intake in people with severe disability is dysphagia (*see* Chapter 18, 'Dysphagia',

p. 154). Psychiatric or behavioural disturbances may also cause reduced or incon-sistent appetite (e.g. in a person with intellectual disability who may not otherwise be able to communicate their feelings, reduced appetite or weight loss may be a symptom of depression).

Underweight is difficult to measure satisfactorily if an accurate height cannot be obtained. However, a marked decrease in subcutaneous fat indicates significant underweight. Serial weight measurements can be an important tool in the assess-ment of underweight and weight loss, and in monitoring the efficacy of therapy. Percentile charts for skinfold thickness can also be used.

Underweight is defined to be a BMI<18.5 kg/m². However, it is not uncommon to find people with severe physical disability to have BMIs in the range of 15 to18. Estimates of the prevalence of underweight vary according to the population stud-ied and the severity of the disability, but up to one-third of people with intellectual disability are thought to be affected. (A nutritional survey of 428 adult and child residents of an institution accommodating people with intellectual disability of various levels revealed that 4.2% were severely underweight [BMI<15] and 8.4% were underweight [BMI 15–18].)

Consequences of underweight

The consequences of underweight may include:
➤ compromised immunity with increased susceptibility to infections
➤ reduced respiratory muscle function
➤ decreased energy levels leading to reduced participation in education, work and social activities
➤ reduced overall quality of life.

If the person also has dysphagia, there may be additional consequences (*see* Chapter 18, 'Dysphagia', p. 154).

Chronic underweight in a person with disability – or in any person – should not be ignored; it has major implications for health.

Assessment

Assessment of underweight in people with intellectual disability often requires a multidisciplinary approach.
➤ Establish the weight (including serial weights if available) and height, or use other measures (such as waist circumference or skinfold thickness).
➤ Look for the cause of underweight (e.g. hyperthyroidism, malignancy, dysphagia, depression).
➤ Check for the presence of associated clinical problems or complications (e.g. aspiration, dehydration, gastro-oesophageal reflux disease, constipation, anaemia, specific micronutrient deficiencies, acute or chronic infection due to reduced immunity).
➤ Refer the patient to a dietician for nutritional assessment and the development of a nutrition care plan.
➤ If dysphagia is present, refer the patient to a speech pathologist for assessment of swallowing, and eating and drinking capabilities; additional investigations may be required (*see* Chapter 18, 'Dysphagia', p. 154).

➤ Refer the patient to an occupational therapist or physiotherapist if assessment of seating (positioning and support) and feeding techniques is required.

➤ Assess the concerns and priorities of all involved individuals, including the person with the developmental disability, family members, other support persons and allied health professionals – this is vital for a collaborative approach to management.

Management

Malnutrition can be insidious in its onset, long-term in nature and apparently resistant to amelioration by obvious remedies such as offering more food. Family members or other support persons sometimes feel that nothing can be done; however, with careful attention to, and patient assistance with, eating and drinking, malnutrition is usually reversible.

1 Thorough assessment is a vital first step.

2 An ethical decision-making framework may assist in making difficult decisions relating to the management of nutritional deficits and dysphagia in people with developmental disability, particularly about providing enteral tube feeds or significantly modifying oral intake. *See* p. 158 for a decision-making framework for the assessment and management of dysphagia.

3 A multidisciplinary approach is also required for management. This can include:

    a A dietician to provide a dietary plan to commence renourishment. This may include supplementing calories and modifying food textures. Commercial products may be used but common foods (such as milk) are often the basis of supplementation. Vitamin and mineral supplements may also be required.

    b A speech pathologist to provide advice regarding feeding techniques and correct positioning (of both the person with the disability and the person assisting with feeding), especially if dysphagia is also present.

4 It may also be necessary to consult:

    a An occupational therapist or seating specialist for seating modification – and advice about seating systems to improve positioning and increase the safety and comfort of the person during mealtimes – especially if dysphagia is also present.

    b A gastroenterologist or respiratory physician to treat associated conditions or complications (e.g. gastro-oesophageal reflux disease, constipation, respiratory infections).

5 Ensure that the person's immunisations are up to date, including influenza and pneumococcal vaccines according to 'The Green Book'. For more information *see* the immunisation section in Chapter 10, 'Preventive Healthcare and Health Promotion' (p. 82).

6 Monitor and regularly review the person's nutritional status and modify the plan as required.

It is crucial to involve all stakeholders in the management plan to ensure its success.

Enteral tube feeding

If the person's poor nutritional status continues, enteral tube feeding (usually by a gastrostomy tube or, if short term, a nasogastric tube) should be considered. A collaborative approach in making this decision involves the person themself, family and other support persons, and the advice of relevant specialists including a dietician, speech pathologist and gastroenterologist. *See also* 'Decision-making framework for the assessment and management of dysphagia' (p. 158). The nutritional goals of tube feeding should be determined before tube feeding commences. The dietician will recommend a liquid formula and the feeding schedule – intermittent bolus or continuous drip. The regimen will likely need a number of adjustments in the short term and periodic monitoring in the longer term to optimise nutritional intake. Support persons need training in managing the equipment; learning the procedures for the administration of formula, other fluids and medications; and care of the gastrostomy site. Stomal therapists or home enteral feeding consulting services can also offer useful assistance in relation to these issues.

Even when their nutritional needs are met completely by enteral tube feeding, some people choose to continue to eat small amounts of certain foods orally for the experience of taste and enjoyment of life.

Enteral tube feeding should not be embarked upon as a long-term treatment for aspiration or chronic chest infections, since it can be associated with risk of aspiration, especially in the presence of gastro-oesophageal reflux disease.

It is important to maintain rigorous oral care routines in the presence of enteral tube feeding, to reduce risks associated with aspiration of saliva and development of respiratory infection.

OVERWEIGHT AND OBESITY

The criteria for defining overweight and obesity in people with developmental disability are much the same as those used in the general population (*see* Tables 17.1 and 17.2, p. 147).

When an accurate height cannot be determined, other measures such as waist circumference or skinfold thickness can be used.

Prevalence

The prevalence of overweight and obesity in people with intellectual disability as cited in the literature varies widely according to the type of population studied, but it is generally accepted to be higher than that of the general community. Most studies show that women, those living in community settings, and people with less severe levels of disability are most at risk. The rates of overweight and obesity in people with Down syndrome are usually higher than for others with intellectual disability. Insufficient physical activity is another major factor contributing to overweight and obesity. People with intellectual disability have higher rates of physical inactivity and lower levels of cardiovascular fitness than are found in the general population.

As with underweight, overweight and obesity are not inevitable in people with intellectual disability. They are usually the result of lifestyle factors and are therefore potentially preventable and treatable. Even in people who have a biological basis to their obesity (e.g. those with Prader-Willi syndrome), it is possible to control weight gain with strict limits to food access.

Consequences of overweight and obesity

People with intellectual disability are just as susceptible to the complications of overweight and obesity as others in the population. These complications include:

➤ coronary artery disease
➤ Type 2 diabetes
➤ hyperlipidaemia
➤ hypertension
➤ obstructive sleep apnoea – people with Down syndrome who tend to have narrow upper airways are especially susceptible
➤ osteoarthritis.

Assessment and management

The assessment and management of overweight and obesity in people with intellectual disability generally follow the same guidelines as for the rest of the population such as the recent NICE guideline. In summary, these guidelines include the following.

➤ Take appropriate anthropometric measurements.
➤ Assess and treat comorbidities.
➤ Assess the nature and causes of energy imbalance.
➤ Ascertain patient motivation to lose weight – in the person with developmental disability, family/support person motivation is equally important.
➤ Determine the level of clinical intervention required.
➤ Devise treatment goals and strategies with the patient (and family/support person in the case of the person with developmental disability).
➤ Prescribe, or refer for advice on, diet and physical activity. (Some clinicians have used both a structured intervention programme – involving a dietician and an exercise physiologist to offer simple dietary advice – and a supervised, group exercise programme. Anecdotal reports show significant weight loss associated with improvement in the individual's self-esteem; other positive health benefits, including improvements in cardiovascular risk factors and increased mobility, were also noted.)
➤ Prescribe medication, or refer for surgery and behaviour modification (as appropriate).
➤ Review and change the programme as required.

Any assessment of overweight and obesity should also include an estimation of the person's physical activity levels, including levels of incidental activity and any barriers to undertaking physical activity.

In people with intellectual disability, additional factors need to be considered and addressed:

➤ Most people with intellectual disability rely on family members or other support persons for their access to food or physical activity. Therefore, the knowledge and attitudes of family members and other support persons to food and dietary intake need to be considered, as well as the goals of the individual with intellectual disability:
 — Support persons (including family members) may have poor knowledge of nutrition and the nutritional needs of the individual with intellectual disability.
 — Overweight and obesity may not be seen as a problem in the person with intellectual disability.

— Food may be used to reward 'good' behaviour or to control unwanted behaviour.
— Food may be used for comfort or as a diversion.
— The notion of 'choice' for the person with intellectual disability may be used as the rationale to allow unlimited access to food.
— Where the person lives in a community setting, the food preferences and nutritional requirements of co-residents may influence the types of food given.
➤ Some individuals with intellectual disability are more physically mobile and independent, and are able to access food independently both inside and outside the home. Cognitive limitations may make educational and behavioural changes more difficult to implement.
➤ Consistency of intervention may be difficult to achieve:
— Different shifts and high turnover of residential staff can lead to inconsistent and sometimes ad hoc decisions about food shopping and meals.
— There are often many settings where intervention needs to be applied (group home, family home, day placement, respite care, social activities).
— Inadequate or inconsistent staffing levels reduce the support available for the person to engage in physical activity.
➤ Other barriers:
— Physical disability may restrict the level of physical activity that a person is able to do.
— Some psychotropic and antiepileptic medications induce weight gain.

Strategies to overcome barriers to losing weight
The following strategies can assist in promoting weight management.
➤ Ensure that family members and key support persons are included in devising management plans.
➤ Refer to a dietician for advice on the individual's diet, food shopping lists and meal plans for the entire household.
➤ Where possible, consider alternative medications that are less likely to cause weight gain.
➤ Consider referring for behavioural intervention to change eating behaviours.
➤ Encourage group-based physical activities so that everyone in the household can participate.

SPECIFIC NUTRITIONAL DEFICIENCIES
Information on the role of vitamin D and calcium in osteoporosis, and vitamin D in osteomalacia can be found in Chapter 8, 'Adult Healthcare' (p. 62).

Vitamin B$_{12}$
Recent research questions the accuracy of currently available laboratory tests for vitamin B$_{12}$ deficiency and suggests that vitamin B$_{12}$ deficiency may be more common than currently recognised. People with intellectual disability may be vulnerable to vitamin B$_{12}$ deficiency due to factors such as:
➤ reduced gastric acid secretion due to gastritis, *Helicobacter pylori* infection or prolonged treatment with acid-inhibiting drugs

➤ gastrointestinal blood loss
➤ coeliac disease (more common in people with Down syndrome).

The symptoms of vitamin B_{12} deficiency include neurological dysfunction. These symptoms can be subtle and difficult to recognise in a person with intellectual disability.

Other nutrient deficiencies

Folate, iron and micronutrient deficiencies may occur in people with undernutrition (e.g. due to dysphagia). These deficiencies should be checked for, and corrected if necessary. Assess vitamin B_{12} status before correcting folate deficiency. People with gastro-oesophageal reflux disease with oesophagitis are especially at risk of iron deficiency due to blood loss.

FURTHER READING

- Bhaumik S, Watson JM, Thorp CF, *et al*. Body mass index in adults with intellectual disability: distribution, associations and service implications: a population-based prevalence study. *J Intellect Disabil Res*. 2008; **52**(4): 287–98.
- Bradford GS, Taylor CT. Omeprazole and vitamin B12 deficiency. *Ann Pharmacother*. 1999; **33**(5): 641–3.
- National institute for Health and Clinical Excellence (NICE). *Guideline CG43: obesity*. NICE; 2010.
- Oh R, Brown DL. Vitamin B12 deficiency. *Am Fam Physician*. 2003; **67**(5): 979–86.

CHAPTER 18

Dysphagia

Dysphagia is common in people with intellectual disability. It has been estimated that its prevalence in adults with multiple disabilities is as high as 76%. People with severe physical disability as a result of cerebral palsy are much more likely to have difficulty in swallowing and possibly malnutrition.

Infants who are diagnosed to have, or who are at risk of having, cerebral palsy or intellectual disability (e.g. extremely low birthweight infants) may also be at risk of having feeding difficulties.

Aspiration pneumonia, commonly associated with dysphagia, is one of the most common causes of death in people with intellectual disability. In a person who has dysphagia and aspiration, eating and drinking without appropriate modifications may be life-threatening. Modifications to dietary intake may prevent people from becoming ill as a result of their difficulty in swallowing. Comprehensive assessment and management are therefore vital.

Some people with intellectual disability experience deterioration in swallowing skills after the age of 30 years that is associated with changes related to ageing. Therefore, it is important to review changes in swallowing ability and oral intake as a person with disability ages.

PRESENTATION

A person with dysphagia and/or aspiration may present with one or several of the following symptoms:
- coughing or choking on food, fluid or saliva
- difficulty with chewing or swallowing – with food or liquid sometimes falling out of the mouth
- taking a long time to eat
- reduction in oral intake
- underweight or weight loss
- chronic wheeze
- recurrent chest infections.

Many symptoms of dysphagia can be observed while the person is having a meal or a drink. However, some symptoms may be less obvious – particularly in those people who have reduced sensation or who do not have an effective or efficient cough reflex. These people may not cough even if they aspirate food, fluid or saliva.

Recommendation

Refer the person to a speech pathologist for full assessment if symptoms of dysphagia are present, or if the person (or their support person) reports any difficulties in swallowing food, fluids or medication.

Consequences of dysphagia can include:
➤ Death from a choking incident.
➤ Aspiration – which may be associated with a number of complications including pneumonia (which can cause death), recurrent respiratory illness, wheezing and night-time coughing. Some of these symptoms may be masked by, or mistaken for, symptoms of asthma; however, they may also be related to aspiration.
➤ Nutritional compromise (malnutrition and dehydration).
➤ Disruptions to normal sensations of hunger and satiety.
➤ A negative impact on psychosocial health (e.g. depression) and social isolation.
➤ Anxiety related to coughing or choking.
➤ Food refusal or food avoidance.
➤ Reduced quality of life.

ASSESSMENT

The assessment of dysphagia may involve a number of professionals and may require both clinical and instrumental investigations. A simple initial screening can be done with checklists such as the Nutrition and Swallowing Checklist (Flintwood Disability Services – www.flintwood.com.au) by either the GP or family member or other support person.

Clinical assessment

Following identification through screening, a comprehensive assessment must be obtained to properly inform decisions regarding interventions for dysphagia. The assessment of dysphagia is multidisciplinary and may include:
➤ The GP – to assess the clinical condition and any associated conditions or complications (e.g. respiratory compromise, gastro-oesophageal reflux disease, malnutrition, oral health problems). An assessment of family and social dynamics, and factors associated with quality of life, is also essential.
➤ The speech pathologist – to make clinical observations on the process of swallowing and symptoms of dysphagia, and to advise on the need for instrumental assessment and the management of the dysphagia.
➤ The dietician – to assess nutritional status and the need for nutritional rehabilitation of the patient, *see also* the section on underweight (p. 147).
➤ Other allied health professionals (e.g. occupational therapist or physiotherapist) – to assess seating and positioning techniques while feeding.

Respiratory physicians and gastroenterologists may also need to be involved for further assessment of the respiratory and gastrointestinal status respectively. The assessment process also needs to involve family members and/or other support persons.

Investigations

The person with dysphagia may also require instrumental investigations such as videofluoroscopy of the swallow (modified barium swallow) or fibre-optic endoscopic examination of the gastro-oesophageal tract. A modified barium swallow result can be used to:

➤ identify the level, degree and type of dysphagia
➤ determine the level and degree of aspiration, and any factors in the swallow contributing to aspiration
➤ assess positioning and other therapeutic strategies that assist in the swallow or that work to reduce the risk or occurrence of aspiration.

Other investigations may include radiology of the chest, and nutritional status tests (e.g. iron studies, full blood count, liver function tests, vitamin B_{12} and folate levels, body composition studies).

MANAGEMENT

The GP should maintain an overview of the dysphagia in relation to other areas of the person's general health and well-being. GPs are equipped to make referrals for instrumental tests (and should consult closely with a speech pathologist to determine which are required) and other investigations. A speech pathologist can also provide information to the GP on the ongoing management of the dysphagia.

Interventions for dysphagia include:

➤ modification of food or fluid consistencies adapted to the difficulty in swallowing – to reduce the risk of aspiration pneumonia and increase efficiency of oral intake
➤ nutritional rehabilitation, if the patient is underweight or is experiencing difficulty in maintaining adequate food intake
➤ oral-motor therapy treatment designed to improve movement of the mouth, lips, tongue and cheeks – to assist in the swallow
➤ design and provision of seating systems – to support the person's posture in the upright position
➤ training of support persons in adaptation of food and fluids
➤ training of support persons in feeding techniques that assist in the swallow
➤ provision of specialised equipment (e.g. cups, spoons) – designed to increase independence or promote a more efficient swallow
➤ alteration to the food quantities, timing or pacing of the meal
➤ use of prompts or reminders regarding a 'safe' swallow (e.g. cough, swallow again, chin down)
➤ management of related health problems (e.g. gastro-oesophageal reflux disease, medications, oral health).

If the patient cannot achieve adequate nourishment despite a reasonable trial of a nutritional care plan, enteral tube feeding should be considered (*see* the section on enteral tube feeding, p. 149). If tube feeding is likely to be longer than four to six weeks, gastrostomy feeding should be considered. Insertion of a gastrostomy tube may be combined with a fundoplication, to reduce gastro-oesophageal reflux and aspiration; however, an individual who has had a gastrostomy with fundoplication may still aspirate oral secretions, so it is important to maintain correct posture and positioning with eating.

Medications

A number of medications can exacerbate dysphagia, either by reducing saliva flow (e.g. anticholinergics), causing nausea, or affecting the neuromotor control of the swallow (e.g. sedatives, psychotropics, antiepileptics). The interaction between medications can also worsen symptoms of dysphagia and interfere with the absorption of nutrients from food. If a person's dysphagia interferes with their ability to take solid-dose oral medications, alternative formulations such as liquid, suppositories or patches can be considered.

Saliva control

Drooling or poor saliva control (sialorrhoea) can be a symptom of difficulty in swallowing, and affects 10% to 37% of people with cerebral palsy, and a significant number of people with Down syndrome. There is a range of surgical, medical and behavioural interventions for saliva management that vary in success. Intervention is interdisciplinary and may include behaviour modification and biofeedback, oromotor therapy, drug therapy and surgery.

Oral health

It is very important that a person with dysphagia follows a rigorous oral care plan to ensure optimal levels of oral health. Poor oral health (resulting in increased levels of bacteria in the oral area) has been implicated as a significant factor in the development of aspiration pneumonia in elderly people who inhale food or fluids. It is important for people with dysphagia and intellectual disability to have a programme of preventive oral care and prompt treatment of dental or gum infections, to reduce the risk of developing respiratory illness related to dysphagia and aspiration. For more information *see* Chapter 19, 'Oral Health' (p. 160).

Seating

The presence of cerebral palsy may impact upon a person's ability to maintain an upright posture for mealtimes or other times of oral intake. Poor posture, or inadequate seating or head support while eating, may contribute to dysphagia and can increase the risk of aspiration. For people with physical disability, a customised seating system may be necessary for optimal positioning during mealtimes, and also for clinical or instrumental assessment of dysphagia and dietary intake. Therefore it is important to consider the person's seating and positioning, and make appropriate referrals (e.g. to an occupational therapist) if the person has difficulty maintaining an upright posture or appropriate head positioning when swallowing.

Communication

People with intellectual disability and dysphagia may also have complex communication needs, and this must be considered and addressed in the assessment and management of dysphagia. *See also* Chapter 4, 'How to Communicate with Your Patient' (p. 29) and Chapter 5, 'Methods of Communication' (p. 34). In order to be included in discussions and decisions relating to their health and mealtimes, people with complex communication needs and dysphagia might require update or redesign of existing forms of augmentative and alternative communication. It is important that a speech pathologist be consulted to determine if a person who is unable to speak might benefit from an augmentative or alternative method of communication, particularly if the person does not have a suitable method for communicating preferences.

Decision-making framework

Box 18.1 presents the decision-making framework for the assessment and management of dysphagia.

BOX 18.1 Decision-making framework for the assessment and management of dysphagia

Identification
- What is the problem?
- Who are the people involved?(consider the individual, family members, guardian, other support persons, health professionals, advocate).
- Who can give consent?

Assessment
(Include clinical assessments – as required, by speech pathologist, dietitian, respiratory physician, gastroenterologist and occupational therapist – and investigations.)
- Swallowing
- Nutrition
- Associated medical conditions
- Complications
- Seating
- Communication
- Quality of life of the individual, family, other support persons

Assess the options for management
- What are the options?
- What are the benefits and risks of each option?
- What are the ethical and legal implications of each option?
- Who and what does each option involve in practical terms?

Make a decision about management
- Consider the values, beliefs and attitudes of all of those involved in the process.
- Take a collaborative approach and choose an option.
- Obtain consent.
- If people can't agree, look for a way to resolve the issue (e.g. conciliation, independent assessment, or as a last resort, application to the Guardianship Tribunal).

Implementation
- Develop a plan to implement the chosen option.
- Implement the plan.
- Monitor, review and amend the plan as appropriate.

FURTHER READING

- Kaatzke-McDonald M. Dysphagia, disability, and icebergs: a discussion. *Adv Speech Lang Pathol.* 2003; **5**(2): 131–5.
- Logemann J. *Evaluation and Treatment of Swallowing Disorders.* 2nd ed. Austin, Texas: Pro-Ed; 1998.
- Patient Safety Agency. Understanding the patient safety issues for people with learning disabilities. 2004. Available at: www.salford-pct.nhs.uk/documents/LD/NPSAUnderstanding.pdf
- Rosenthal S, Sheppard JJ, Lotze M. *Dysphagia in the Child with Developmental Disabilities: medical, clinical and family interventions.* San Diego, CA: Singular Publishing Group; 1995.
- Sheppard JJ. Managing dysphagia in mentally retarded adults. *Dysphagia.* 1991; **6**(2): 83–7.
- Sonies BC. *Dysphagia: a continuum of care.* Gaithersburg, Maryland: Aspen; 1996.

CHAPTER 19

Oral health

People with intellectual disability are at considerable risk of developing dental disease. The effect of poor oral health on general health has been well documented. Poor oral health increases the risk of aspiration pneumonia, complicates the management of diabetes and is a risk factor for heart disease. Furthermore, nutritional status is greatly affected by oral health status.

Factors that increase the risk of dental disease in people with intellectual disability include:

➤ inadequate plaque removal
➤ a reliance on support persons, who may find it difficult to deliver adequate oral care due to the challenging behaviour of the people with developmental disability
➤ the person's diet, which may include frequent ingestion of small meals and drinks that are high in sugars and other carbohydrates
➤ poor oral clearance of foodstuff (leaving food debris around the teeth)
➤ drug-induced xerostomia (dry mouth)
➤ excessive salivation – often resulting from oropharyngeal deformity but sometimes of no definite cause
➤ an increased incidence of gastro-oesophageal reflux disease.

Patient fear can be a barrier to providing optimal dental care or performing oral examinations. Using a person's own toothbrush (instead of a spatula) may facilitate inspecting the mouth of a person with intellectual disability. Some people are sufficiently traumatised by oral examinations that they require the administration of a sedative or general anaesthetic for examinations or treatment to take place.

DENTAL CARIES (TOOTH DECAY)

Saliva prevents tooth decay by washing food debris away. It also remineralises teeth by charging them with calcium and phosphate ions. People with intellectual disability are frequently on medications that cause a dry mouth and thus are more likely to experience dental decay.

Consider the following strategies to reduce the incidence of tooth decay:

➤ Provide saliva substitutes (which replace missing enzymes such as lactoperoxidase, lactoferin and lysozyme) for people with xerostomia.

➤ Advise people with xerostomia to use high-dose fluoride toothpaste.
➤ Educate people with intellectual disability (and their support persons) to brush with fluoride toothpaste twice a day.
➤ Discourage the frequent consumption of high carbohydrate snacks and sugary drinks.
➤ Provide healthy alternative snacks, such as cheese and nuts.
➤ Provide alternative sweet foods such as lollies that are sweetened with xylitol (these should be consumed in moderation to avoid osmotic diarrhoea).
➤ Promote the consumption of water between meals.

DENTAL EROSION (TOOTH WEAR)

Gastro-oesophageal reflux disease introduces stomach acid into the oral cavity at regular intervals. The acid erodes the teeth, leaving them hypersensitive. The degree and pattern of tooth wear may be the first indicators that people suffer from GORD. The management of tooth wear is complex. In severe cases, the entire dentition requires restoration using an overlay technique that is both expensive and complex. Early diagnosis of GORD is essential to avoid the need for restorations.

PERIODONTAL DISEASE (GUM DISEASE)

People with intellectual disability may demonstrate challenging behaviours during the tooth brushing event. If used incorrectly, a toothbrush can cause trauma to soft tissues of the mouth, and people naturally resist tooth brushing if they have been traumatised by it in the past. Failure to clean teeth effectively will result in periodontal disease, which results in tooth loss as the supportive structures of teeth resorb.

All people with intellectual disability require some assistance to clean their teeth, as it is a complex process requiring a combination of fine motor skills and planning.

Brushing a person's teeth can be a complex task, and support persons require training in how to brush people's teeth satisfactorily, in a manner that causes no discomfort.

People with Down syndrome are more susceptible to periodontal disease (due to reduced immunologic response brought about by neutropenia), and thorough tooth brushing and interdental cleaning is imperative.

DENTAL MALOCCLUSION

People with intellectual disability have an increased incidence of oromotor dysfunction. The failure of the facial muscles to function effectively increases the likelihood of people developing a dental malocclusion. Conventional orthodontics may not be possible for patients with challenging behaviours. To obtain the best result, appropriate management is needed as the malocclusion is developing.

EXCESSIVE SALIVATION AND DRIBBLING

Excessive salivation can lead to increased dental decay, severe halitosis and distress due to intertrigo and other skin soreness resulting from dribbling. This can be reduced by correcting neck posture with 'splinting' in the form of woolly scarves, but if not a trial of hyoscine patches can produce considerable benefit.

FURTHER READING

- Finkelstein DM, Crysdale WS. Evaluation and management of the drooling patient. *J Otolaryngol.* 1992; **21**(6): 414–18.
- Holland TJ, O'Mullane DM. The organisation of dental care for groups of mentally handicapped persons. *Community Dent Health.* 1990; **7**(3): 285–93.
- Langmore SE, Terpenning MS, Schork A, *et al.* Predictors of aspiration pneumonia: how important is dysphagia? *Dysphagia.* 1998; **13**(2): 69–81.

CHAPTER 20

Sexuality

People with intellectual disability have the same variety of sexual desires and needs as the rest of the community. There are many myths surrounding the sexuality of people with intellectual disability. They are often seen either as asexual and childlike and in need of protection, or conversely as oversexed and in danger of becoming promiscuous, perverted or sex offenders. Neither view holds up to scrutiny. There are differences, however, but these have more to do with different life experiences and opportunities to learn, rather than the individual's inherent sexuality. It is by acknowledging and acting upon these differences that people with intellectual disability can be best assisted to develop to their full potential.

There are many aspects to human sexuality and only a few of the most common will be discussed here. Sexuality and disability is often considered a Pandora's box of complex and never-ending problems. It is important to:

➤ treat the person with the same amount of respect and dignity as you would a person with no disability
➤ be respectful, not only of the person but also of their disability
➤ consider as a starting point what treatment or counselling you would provide if this person did not have a disability
➤ be aware of myths and stereotypes
➤ consider what is the function or purpose of the behaviour.

FACTORS AFFECTING DEVELOPMENT OF SEXUALITY

There are a number of factors affecting what people with intellectual disability experience and learn about their sexuality. These factors may affect knowledge of basic body parts or diseases, appropriate social and sexual behaviour, and appropriate expression of sexual needs and sexuality; or they may influence behaviour. For example, public masturbation may be the result of a lack of understanding of the differences between public and private places and behaviours rather than a desire to be sexually perverse.

Social factors

Information about sexuality is generally acquired through life experiences. For people with intellectual disability, these may be overseen by others or be limited because of the disability. People with intellectual disability often have difficulty learning and generalising the abstract social rules and patterns of behaviour that govern our society; they also may learn inappropriate behaviours from others, both with and without disabilities.

Access to information

People with intellectual disability do not have the same access to information about sexuality as people without disability have, including formal education, easy-to-read literature and access to appropriate generic agencies.

Factors relating to specific disabilities

People with autism may have problems understanding the basic concepts of social interaction. Those with sensory impairments may have limited opportunities to experience pleasure. People with limited communication skills may have reduced opportunities to interact with others.

COUNSELLING

It is important to provide people with intellectual disability and those supporting them with appropriate and accessible information on sexuality, and how the individual can incorporate this part of their identity into their daily lives. Doctors play a substantial role as educators. The appropriate approach to these problems will vary according to the needs of each patient.

Most people with intellectual disability experience some difficulty when dealing with concepts that are abstract; explanations must be specific.
➤ Keep language simple and concrete.
➤ Repeat what is said.
➤ Demonstrate wherever possible. Use simple and clear pictures, realistic models or the actual object. Demonstrate using the person's own body (as appropriate).
➤ Check and recheck that the person has understood. Rephrase and ask the same questions in different ways to check that the person has understood the information or instructions.

ISSUES OF PRIVACY

People with intellectual disability do not experience the same degree of privacy as people without disability.

For example, a young man with intellectual disability may wish to masturbate and look at sexually explicit magazines in the privacy of his bedroom. If he lives in a house supervised by support workers with access to his bedroom, the magazines may be discovered and various restrictions and interventions imposed. If this young man did not have intellectual disability probably no one would know. However, even if it was known:
➤ it would probably not be considered unusual or abnormal behaviour requiring intervention
➤ the young man would probably be able to assert his right to privacy.

INAPPROPRIATE SEXUAL BEHAVIOUR

Inappropriate sexual behaviour may be due to lack of knowledge or lack of experience, or be related to a person's disability. For example, a propensity to repetitive and obsessive behaviour may impact on the patient's expression of their sexuality, and difficult or unusual behaviours may manifest in a sexual manner (e.g. chronic constipation leading to anal masturbation).

If inappropriate sexual behaviours occur, exclude the underlying medical and/ or psychiatric causes and refer for behavioural management and education (if appropriate).

When counselling a person who demonstrates inappropriate sexual behaviour:

➤ consider the underlying cause of their disability and the associated problems
➤ encourage ongoing education in all aspects of human relations and sexuality – a number of agencies provide this education (e.g. disability services departments can provide information, *see* p. 255)
➤ encourage the person to seek opportunities to develop worthwhile and meaningful relationships (including sexual relationships) with others.

MASTURBATION

Masturbation is a normal and natural experience for men and women in all age ranges. At times, masturbation may not in itself be a sexual act but purely a means of sensory stimulation that the person has learnt is readily accessible and usually pleasurable. Masturbation at the appropriate time and place is usually acceptable behaviour.

Encourage acceptable behaviour by:

➤ redirecting the person to their room when appropriate
➤ ensuring privacy at this time
➤ ensuring age-appropriate access to materials such as magazines, posters and pictures
➤ providing appropriate education and opportunities to explore this aspect of their sexual development
➤ teaching socially acceptable rules of sexual behaviour (i.e. masturbation is an activity that occurs in a private place such as a bedroom)
➤ educating support persons in what is socially acceptable behaviour, if necessary.

Excessive masturbation

Parents and other support persons may become concerned when the frequency of the masturbation is excessive. Just what is excessive is often a moot point. If it results in physical injury or impacts significantly on normal daily life, a cause should be looked for. Usually, there is no medical cause; it is often the result of boredom and lack of other meaningful and enjoyable activities.

Changing environmental factors often impacts on the frequency of masturbation. Redirecting the person to other activities may be the most appropriate strategy for support persons.

Anal masturbation

A number of people derive sexual pleasure from anal masturbation. This is sometimes associated with faecal smearing. If this is how a person has chosen to masturbate, it is quite likely that they will continue with this practice despite how others feel. It is therefore important that they are encouraged to be responsible in this practice.

Responsible practices include:
➤ no faecal smearing
➤ good hygiene habits both before and after masturbation
➤ that foreign objects and sex toys used during masturbation are unbreakable, have smooth surfaces and can be retrieved
➤ that it is always a private activity.

HOMOSEXUALITY

There is no reason to suggest that homosexuality occurs with any more or less frequency in people with intellectual disability than it does in the rest of the population. However, as many older people with intellectual disability have spent long periods of their lives in institutions, usually living in same-sex units, their experiences may have been limited to same-sex sexual activity. Rather than this being a sexual preference, it may have been brought about by limited and restricted opportunities to engage in a wider range of sexual experiences.

Recommendation

➤ Ensure individuals have opportunities to socialise and experience a range of relationships in order to help them more fully understand their own sexual preferences.
➤ Emphasise safe sexual practices.

SEXUAL ABUSE AND EXPLOITATION

One of the main concerns of parents and other support persons of people with intellectual disability is their greater degree of vulnerability to sexual abuse and exploitation. People with intellectual disability are more likely to be sexually abused because they:
➤ often do not understand what is happening to them
➤ are less able to protect themselves
➤ are unlikely to report abuse
➤ are less likely to be believed even if they do report sexual abuse.

Sexual abuse is common in people with intellectual disability and it is essential to follow through if complaints and allegations of abuse are made. It is important to assess if the alleged victim is able to give informed consent for sexual activity. The power differential between the alleged perpetrator and the victim will give an indication of whether abuse or exploitation has occurred.

In responding to suspicions or disclosure of sexual abuse, deal with allegations of abuse in the same way as for a person without disability. This may include referral to an appropriate sexual abuse counselling agency.

SEXUAL OFFENDING BEHAVIOUR

Men with intellectual disability are often seen to be perpetrators of sexual abuse and/or sexual exploitation. However, this occurs per percentage of population with no more frequency than it does within the rest of the community. As with non-disabled offenders, there are multiple social influences that result in a person with intellectual disability becoming a sexual offender. Sex offending is not the result of a high sex drive.

It is essential to refer people suspected of perpetrating sexual abuse for specialist treatment; also to ensure that the alleged abuse is reported to the appropriate authorities. Although treatment options for people with disability have been limited in the past, treatment approaches and services have begun to be developed. Treatment should include social, psychological, educational, medical and psychiatric aspects.

It is inappropriate to prescribe antiandrogens (e.g. medroxyprogesterone and cyproterone) to curtail sexual libido simply because the person is perceived by others to have a problem with their sexuality. If such medication is warranted and the person is unable to give informed consent, permission must be obtained under the terms of the Mental Capacity Act from the relative or carer acting on the patient's behalf.

CONTRACEPTION

It is important to remind people that although providing contraception may remove the fear of an unwanted pregnancy, it does not lessen or diminish vulnerability to sexual abuse, exploitation or sexually transmissible infections (STIs). Parents or other support persons of people with intellectual disability may be anxious when the person in their care becomes sexually active. This anxiety may be an over-reaction to the risks and the vulnerability of the person and each case needs to be assessed on its merits.

When considering contraception for people with intellectual disability, assess the needs of the individual from the least restrictive point of view and not what may be easier for parents or other support persons. Explore the views of the person with intellectual disability. If possible spend time talking directly to them. Many people with mild to moderate degrees of intellectual disability can cope with the oral contraceptive pill.

Whatever contraceptive choice is made it should always include:
➤ education, information and discussion around the rights and responsibilities of being sexually active
➤ discussion of protective behaviour strategies and safe sex practices, including safe touching, as well as the use of condoms.

Consider informing parents or other support persons of the timing and types of appropriate medical review, and the potential adverse effects of the chosen contraception.

See also Chapter 21, 'Women's Health' (p. 171).

STERILISATION

Although relatively simple, operations such as sterilisation procedures, including endometrial ablation and vasectomy need consent to be obtained according to the Mental Capacity Act. Sterilisation procedures should only be considered for the same therapeutic reasons as for anyone else. *See also* Chapter 23, 'Legal Issues' (p. 183).

PREVENTIVE HEALTHCARE

The usual range of preventive healthcare measures that are offered to others in the community should also be considered for people with intellectual disability.

Education about STIs is necessary for people who are or may be sexually active, and should be provided at the appropriate learning level in conjunction with appropriate health screening. Some preventive health measures may require physical examination and it is important to take the time to familiarise the patient with exactly what is going to happen during the procedure. This may be done over several visits. It may also help if someone that the person feels comfortable with is present and offers support during the physical examination.

Occasionally, performing the procedure would cause excessive distress to the patient. Some procedures need to be performed under general anaesthetic; the risks and benefits involved require careful consideration first.

FURTHER READING

- Mitchell L. *Normalisation and Sexuality of the Mentally Handicapped*. Thomas Publishers; 1985.
- Ross MW, Channon-Little LD. *Discussing Sexuality: a guide for health practitioners*. Sydney: Maclennan and Petty; 1991.

CHAPTER 21

Women's health

The management of health issues in women with intellectual disability should be approached in the same way as for women in the general population. Successful management requires being aware of the complex issues related to sexual and reproductive health in women with intellectual disability, and the need for appropriate support resources to assist education, counselling and clinical treatment.

MANAGEMENT PRINCIPLES

Clinical management of women's health issues involves a complex interaction of issues relating to:
➤ patient and support person knowledge of, and attitudes to, menstruation, sexuality and disability
➤ hygienic menstrual management
➤ fertility control
➤ real or perceived needs for protection from sexual abuse
➤ preventive care measures
➤ informed consent
➤ availability of support resources.

Management should be guided by the following principles.
➤ Women with intellectual disability have the right to current standards of care and the full range of management options.
➤ The woman's best interests are the highest priority, rather than the interests of others.
➤ Education strategies are seen as the first stage of the continuum of least restrictive alternatives.
➤ There is an obligation to overcome physical, cognitive and communication difficulties.

MENARCHE AND ONSET OF PUBERTY

Recent rigorous research is limited but indicates menarchal age is not usually delayed in women with intellectual disability. However, early menstrual cycles most often follow a similar pattern to the general population.

Delayed puberty is rarely associated with the primary aetiology of the disability.

However, low bodyweight due to problems associated with the disability may delay puberty.

Recommendation

➤ Investigate if menarche has not occurred by age 16 (as in the general population).
➤ Consider low bodyweight and poor nutrition in association with the investigation of delayed menarche (both of which also may impact adversely on bone density development).

MENSTRUAL MANAGEMENT

As it is for all women, the aim of menstrual management for the woman with intellectual disability is that she understands and manages a normal body function in a hygienic and socially acceptable manner, with assistance where necessary.

Acquiring self-care skills and so identifying with the normal female population is an essential part of developing self-esteem. Carers or supporting family should report a menstrual history at the time of annual health checks.

Education

Specific education assists the majority of women with intellectual disability to manage their own personal hygiene with or without supervision. Women with severe intellectual disability can be encouraged to be involved in, or tolerant of, assistance with hygienic menstrual management.

Recommendation

➤ Explain about menstruation repeatedly and directly (e.g. as bleeding that all women have each month from a hole between their legs).
➤ Teach pad management by demonstrating on the woman's body (the preferable method), imitating, or using an anatomically correct doll. If pads can't be tolerated, demonstrate the use of products developed for incontinence management.
➤ Teach the private nature of menstruation.

The instruction process should begin before menarche to avoid the occurrence of inappropriate behaviour (such as menstrual blood smearing), which has been suggested as more likely if no menstrual preparation has occurred.

Teaching resources for menstrual management are available through a number of organisations. Many family planning associations offer programmes for people with intellectual disability.

REPRODUCTION
Education

Education regarding sex and interpersonal relationships may need to be modified according to the individual's capabilities; they should not be delayed, however, as physical maturational rates are most likely to be normal and sexual awareness present.

GPs can often provide useful advice to family members and other support persons about appropriate resources available, and can directly talk with and assist in educating the individual.

Sexuality

Sexual intercourse and pregnancy are least likely in the most severely disabled women who may, however, express their sexuality by masturbating or by other sexual behaviours.

Women with mild intellectual disability are more likely to be sexually active than women with severe intellectual disability; they are also reported to be at greater risk of sexual abuse than those with more severe disability.

Pregnancy outcomes

Pregnancy outcomes suggest a 40% to 50% risk of intellectual disability in progeny of Down syndrome mothers and parents with IQ less than 80, compared to the 1% risk in the general population. This may be related to both genetic and social factors influencing parenting competence.

Parents with intellectual disability are frequently socially isolated and poorly supported by community and personal networks. Parenting capacity should not be presumed to be inadequate, however, and strengthening social support systems in such families is likely to be associated with better outcomes.

HEALTH SCREENING

The principles and practice of women's health screening procedures are the same as for the general population. Often practical difficulties (e.g. in doing mammograms, vaginal examinations and Pap smears) can be overcome by reassuring, explaining, and using appropriate educational aids to prepare the patient for the procedure. Breast cancer is more common and cervical cancer less common in the population. A patient's refusal to undergo these tests must not exclude her from the rest of an annual check. In Glasgow it has been estimated that if every woman with intellectual disability was screened less than 1.4 cases of cervical cancer per annum would be detected – annual health checks have a dramatically higher detection rate for other disorders.

There is a high incidence of sexual abuse in adults with intellectual disability. If abuse is suspected it should be addressed.

Recommendation

➤ Perform two-yearly cervical screening (Pap smear) for women aged 18 to 70 years who have any history of sexual activity and can give consent.
➤ If the examination is distressing or difficult, the risks of a Pap smear (with or without sedation or anaesthesia) need to be balanced against the benefits. Patients with severe adductor spasm due to cerebral palsy and those with severe spinal abnormalities find the procedure particularly distressing.
➤ Mammography, two-yearly after the age of 50 years. In the UK patients with physical disabilities often cannot cope with access to and conditions in the mobile screening units and so provision needs to be provided in the larger, usually hospital-based centres.
➤ Regular breast examination by a GP (frequency not clearly established).

CONTRACEPTION

In addition to contraceptive advice, the following need to be addressed:

➤ teaching about relationships and protection from STIs, especially the use of condoms
➤ education about the right to say 'no'.

The person's ability to give informed consent needs to be assessed.

As contraception diminishes the potential consequence of pregnancy, by removing this consequence, the risk of sexual abuse or STIs may increase.

The full range of options for contraception is available to women with intellectual disability, but the choice of options may be limited by the woman's:

➤ intellectual capacity (partner's capability may be relevant)
➤ physical manipulative skills (partner's capability may be relevant)
➤ social skills
➤ medical conditions, physical disabilities and medication.

Requirements for contraception can be assessed, and methods taught with patience, understanding and appropriate specific counselling. The method chosen should be the best available for the woman, not necessarily the easiest to provide.

Rhythm method and barrier methods

The correct, effective use of the rhythm method (periodic abstinence) and barrier methods is difficult to teach and their use is rarely found to be suitable for women with intellectual disability. Occasionally, a less disabled partner can overcome some difficulties. Significant failure rates of these methods (approximately 15% to 20%) must be considered, together with the lack of protection from STIs.

Combined oral contraception

Effectiveness of oral contraception depends on compliance. Many women with intellectual disability can be reliable pill takers or can be partially or totally assisted (or supervised) by their support persons.

Coincident disabilities may be contraindications (e.g. immobility, past cardiovascular accidents and deep vein thrombosis). Clinical experience also suggests that the oral contraceptive pill may aggravate very unstable epilepsy, particularly if seizure frequency is related to the menstrual cycle. Well-controlled epilepsy is not a contraindication to the use of the oral contraceptive pill.

Drug interactions can occur. Phenytoin, carbamazepine, phenobarbitone and primidone induce hepatic microsomal enzymes metabolising oestrogen and increase the levels of sex-hormone-binding globulin, thereby decreasing oestrogen plasma levels, producing breakthrough bleeding and contraceptive failure. Sodium valproate, vigabatrin and lamotrigine do not interact with the oral contraceptive pill.

Recommendation

➤ Use a pill containing ethinyloestradiol 50 micrograms in women taking phenytoin, carbamazepine, phenobarbitone or primidone, and reduce the pill-free interval to four or five days.
➤ Using a higher dose pill (maximum ethinyloestradiol 80 to 100 micrograms) possibly prevents the occurrence of breakthrough bleeding.

Progestogen-only contraception

Progestogen-only contraception is effective and valuable if oestrogen is contraindicated. Good compliance is essential with the progestogen-only pill.

DEPOT MEDROXYPROGESTERONE ACETATE (DMPA)

Depot medroxyprogesterone acetate is an option when regular pill taking is difficult. It has advantages of extremely effective long-term contraception with a low incidence of adverse effects, no known drug interactions, protection against pelvic inflammatory disease, endometrial and ovarian carcinoma, and the production of amenorrhoea. Adverse effects reported for DMPA include weight gain, depression, mood change and headache. There is no evidence from long-term follow-up studies of increased risk of breast cancer. Menses can take on average four to six months to return to a normal pattern after its use, and conception can be delayed as long as 18 months.

There is potential for the drug to be misused in women who cannot give informed consent to its use or to sexual intercourse. A careful discussion of its use is mandatory with those responsible for the woman's care.

ETONOGESTREL SUBDERMAL IMPLANT

Etonogestrel subdermal implant is an extremely effective and convenient form of contraception and is another option when compliance is an issue. Insertion and removal is a simple office procedure done under local anaesthetic. Most (80% to 85%) users have periods that are similar to or less frequent than their previous cycle pattern, but 15% to 20% of users may have more frequent, sometimes protracted, periods. An etonogestrel implant may not be appropriate if an unpredictable bleeding pattern is unacceptable. It does not affect bone mineral density, and its effects on ovarian function rapidly reverse after removal. The manufacturer cautions against its concomitant use with drugs that induce liver microsomal enzymes.

Intrauterine devices (IUDs)

Intrauterine devices are generally not appropriate in women with intellectual disability, as there can be difficulties related to insertion, follow-up checks of correct placement, as well as possible delays in detecting symptoms related to complications. Menstruation is also likely to be heavier and more painful with the use of IUDs, but menstrual loss is markedly reduced with the newly available levonorgestrel-containing IUS. This expensive device significantly reduces menstrual blood loss and menstrual pain and can produce amenorrhoea in a minority (10% to 20%) of women depending on its duration of use. Its insertion, however, may present difficulties for women with intellectual disability and often will need general anaesthesia.

Sterilisation

Sterilisation may be an option as a form of contraception if it is in the woman's best interests and other less restrictive and reversible methods of contraception are unable to be used or have been trialled and found unsatisfactory. However, there is legislation about when sterilisation may occur and consent needs to be obtained under the terms of the Mental Capacity Act from the patient or carer or responsible member of the family. For more information, *see* Chapter 23, 'Legal Issues' (p. 183).

Emergency contraception

For emergency contraception, use levonorgestrel as a single dose.

Ongoing contraception should be considered and the risk of STIs reviewed. There is no medical contraindication to this form of emergency contraception and it is available over the counter from pharmacists, though it is cheaper on prescription.

MENOPAUSE

Menopause tends to be at an earlier age than average, particularly in women with Down syndrome. In women with Down syndrome, menopause occurs four to five years earlier than average and is independent of the increased tendency to hypothyroidism in these women. Troublesome menopausal symptoms may not be reported or observed in women with developmental disability and should be actively sought at the annual health check.

Multiple risk factors for osteoporosis and cardiovascular disease occur frequently in women with intellectual disability. The incidence of these diseases has been reported as being higher in women with intellectual disability than the general population.

Recommendation

➤ Consider general measures including attention to low-fat diets with adequate calcium, vitamin D status and maintenance of cardiovascular fitness as far as possible.
➤ Assess bone mineral density, if appropriate, where risk factors are present.
➤ Use hormone replacement therapy as in the general population for management of menopausal symptoms, and prophylaxis for women at significant risk of osteoporosis and in whom the benefits of hormone therapy outweigh risk.

GYNAECOLOGICAL PROBLEMS

The principles guiding the management of gynaecological problems in women with intellectual disability should be the same as in women in the general population. Women with intellectual disability are entitled to the full range of management options and the same standards of care as women in the general population, and there is an obligation on the part of the practitioner to attempt as far as possible to overcome difficulties encountered in the delivery of such care.

➤ Gynaecological problems can present particular difficulties in diagnosis, as history details may not be easily obtained either from the woman or her support persons.
➤ Pelvic examination may be difficult to perform and interpret, or not possible at all without an anaesthetic. Ultrasound may help clarify the clinical picture but is usually limited to abdominal ultrasound.
➤ Menstrual charting is often useful.
➤ Symptoms indicating pathology warrant examination under anaesthesia if satisfactory examination cannot be achieved.

Menstrual problems

The incidence of menstrual disorders in women with intellectual disability is difficult to assess and is rarely reported. Clinical experience would suggest that the spectrum of problems is the same as seen in the general population.

Adolescent menstrual irregularity, menorrhagia and dysmenorrhoea

Menstrual irregularity, menorrhagia (heavy periods) and dysmenorrhoea (painful periods) are common during adolescence in all women. Using NSAIDs (to reduce dysmenorrhoea and heavy bleeding) or the contraceptive pill (to produce regular light periods with less dysmenorrhoea) may help. Dysmenorrhoea (and premenstrual syndrome [PMS]) may present as cyclic problematic behaviour. Prospective charting of behaviour can confirm such a relationship and appropriate specific treatment be given.

Oligomenorrhoea

Oligomenorrhoea (infrequent periods) appears to be common in women with intellectual disability, particularly in those who are underweight or overweight. It is often related to other medical conditions or medication.

Menstrual disturbances, polycystic ovary syndrome and hyperandrogenism

Menstrual disturbances, polycystic ovary syndrome and hyperandrogenism are seen more commonly in women with epilepsy, which is frequently associated with intellectual disability. These disorders are possibly more common in women taking sodium valproate and may be an effect of the drug, although the mechanism is unclear.

Hyperprolactinaemia and secondary amenorrhoea

Some major tranquillisers (e.g. phenothiazines and butyrophenones) are well-known to produce hyperprolactinaemia and secondary amenorrhoea. (*See* Chapter 15, 'Management of Psychiatric Disorders', p. 121.)

Premenstrual syndrome

As in the general population, disturbed behaviour related to the menstrual cycle can be due to premenstrual syndrome or dysmenorrhoea. In women with intellectual disability, this may be associated with self-injury.

The relationship between disturbed behaviour and menstruation needs to be charted for three cycles, as behavioural change is often related to other factors and not to PMS (as in the general population also). Charts need to be developed to address individual symptomatology.

Management is along the same lines as for all women (i.e. providing explanations and extra support during stressful times).

Treatment options include pyridoxine (vitamin B_6) 50 to 100 mg orally, daily; evening primrose oil 1 to 3 g orally, daily in the luteal phase; suppression of ovulation with the contraceptive pill; and luteal phase progestogen. None of these therapies has proved to be better than placebo in controlled trials.

Antidepressant therapy with fluoxetine 20 mg orally, daily or for 14 days of the luteal phase of the cycle, has been shown to be effective in placebo-controlled trials. These results may justify its use. However, optimum duration of use for effectiveness is not yet established, and there is potential for interaction with other prescribed psychoactive medication.

MENSTRUAL SUPPRESSION

Menstrual suppression is the temporary or permanent cessation of menstruation by the use of pharmacologically active substances or surgical intervention.

There are some medical and behaviour management problems where menstrual suppression is in the best interests of the woman but this should only be considered when all less restrictive options have been trialled and failed.

Conditions and situations where menstrual suppression may be appropriate include gynaecological conditions (such as menorrhagia, endometriosis and PMS), catamenial (menstrual-associated) epilepsy, when it is an informed decision or request of the woman, and when a woman is likely to injure herself or others.

Decisions to use medication to suppress menstruation solely because of behaviour problems are controversial and best made by a multidisciplinary group in conjunction with the support persons/carers of the woman. *See* Chapter 23, 'Legal Issues' (p. 183).

Continuous progestogens

Until recently, norethisterone was widely used in institutions:
➤ norethisterone 5 mg orally, daily.

Reports of observed adverse effects are few, but the long-term effects are uncertain. Reservations have been expressed about using norethisterone, particularly in women older than 35 years, after an increased incidence of coronary atheroma was reported in long-term users.

Medroxyprogesterone acetate (MPA) is used in the treatment of endometriosis:
➤ medroxyprogesterone acetate (MPA) 10 mg orally, twice daily.

This dose of MPA is associated with a significant incidence of PMS-like adverse effects and breakthrough bleeding in women in the general population.

Oral contraceptive pill

The tricyclic regimen of 12 weeks of hormone tablets (four consecutive 21-day packs of monophasic contraceptive pills) followed by a seven-day break will produce amenorrhoea for 12 weeks followed by a withdrawal bleed. Although there can be some breakthrough bleeding, this regimen usually reduces the number of menses to three or four a year, and associated problems may be more manageable.

It is considered by most, but not proved, that the benefit of the pill-free interval in the contraceptive pill, while associated with withdrawal bleeding, is that it allows pill-affected lipid and coagulation values to return to normal. Thus it is not recommended that it is taken continuously for more than 12 weeks.

Injectable progestogens

Depot medroxyprogesterone acetate (DMPA) (Depo Provera, Depo Ralovera) produces amenorrhoea in 30% of users in three months and in 50% after 12 months:
➤ depot medroxyprogesterone acetate (DMPA) 150 mg IM, 12-weekly.

DMPA has also been reported to reduce seizure frequency in catamenial epilepsy. Most studies report no adverse effects on lipids. DMPA may have a long-term small adverse effect on bone mineral density, which is reversible when discontinued. If

DMPA is used for longer than five years, monitor bone mineral density and, if low, consider stopping DMPA, particularly if there are other significant risk factors for osteoporosis.

Surgery

Surgical procedures for the management of menstruation are not often required and should only be considered after trials of education and medical approaches.

Endometrial ablation

Endometrial ablation has been proposed as a less restrictive surgical option than hysterectomy to eliminate menstruation. Endometrial ablation produces amenorrhoea in about 50% and oligomenorrhoea in about 30%. With time menstruation returns, and about 30% require further surgery in five years. Endometrial ablation does not result in guaranteed infertility.

Hysterectomy

Hysterectomy to eliminate normal menstruation is rarely appropriate and almost never justified prior to the menarche.

The only long-term adverse effect related to hysterectomy with ovarian conservation is a possible lowering of menopausal age by three to four years. This is possibly due to an alteration in ovarian blood flow. If bilateral salpingo-oophorectomy is performed at the time of hysterectomy, a surgically induced menopause will occur which is often distressingly symptomatic and in the longer term is associated with increased risk of coronary artery disease and osteoporosis.

FURTHER READING

- Grover SR. Menstrual and contraceptive management in women with an intellectual disability. *Med J Aust.* 2002; **176**(3): 108–10.

CHAPTER 22

Men's health

Men with intellectual disability have the right to, and should receive, identical healthcare to that of men in the general population unless there is a clear and explicit reason for deviating from this standard – and the reasons for deviations from standard care should be documented.

This chapter highlights the differences in management of men's health issues that are the result of intellectual disability.

Men with intellectual disability may experience some benefits in their health compared to the general population. In the general population, specific health issues for men (apart from those related to male-specific organs) include a propensity for increased risk taking (particularly in younger men), and a reluctance to seek healthcare (especially preventive). Men with more severe levels of intellectual disability are:

➤ less likely to smoke or drink alcohol (and those who do, smoke less and drink less than their counterparts in the general population), which has a positive impact on their cardiovascular risk
➤ unlikely to reach the same degree of risk taking as is the general population; however, the consequences in those who suffer trauma may be greater because of their underlying disability
➤ likely to have more frequent access to routine and preventive healthcare, as this is generally organised by support persons.

When managing the health of men with intellectual disability some problems can be anticipated. Many endocrine diseases (such as androgen deficiency) present with a predominance of symptoms rather than physical signs. People with intellectual disability may not present with symptoms but in an atypical fashion – because they have difficulties communicating verbally. A high degree of clinical suspicion and regular surveillance is required.

ANDROGEN DEFICIENCY

Androgen deficiency has a prevalence of 1 in 200 men. It is more common in men with intellectual disability (particularly men with Down syndrome), where it is less likely to be recognised or, if recognised, less likely to be formally acknowledged. Untreated androgen deficiency is compatible with a long but impoverished quality of life. It may be under-diagnosed due to its subtle and variable clinical features. It may result from hyperprolactinaemia as the result of neuroleptic or other medication (*see* Chapter 15, 'Management of Psychiatric Disorders', p. 121).

Symptoms
Symptoms of androgen deficiency are different depending on the age when the deficiency is detected.

Early teenage years
Symptoms may show in the early teenage years as failure to undergo normal pubertal development. This may manifest as failure of:
➤ the penis and testes to grow
➤ facial, body and pubic hair to appear
➤ the voice to deepen
➤ increased muscle development
➤ the growth surge seen at this time.

There may also be gynaecomastia (although this is not uncommon in normal pubertal development).

Adult years
In adult life, many symptoms are non-specific and include:
➤ increased fatigability and decreased energy
➤ altered mood
➤ irritability
➤ poor concentration
➤ loss of interest in sex and problems achieving erections
➤ hot flushes
➤ gynaecomastia
➤ osteoporosis.

Many people with these symptoms will not be androgen-deficient.

Diagnosis
The diagnosis is made by measuring serum testosterone and luteinising hormone levels, and it is suggested that values of:
➤ less than 8 nanomoles/L are diagnostic of androgen deficiency (independent of the luteinising hormone level)
➤ 8 to 15 nanomoles/L are indeterminate (unless the luteinising hormone value is high, when a diagnosis of androgen deficiency is confirmed)
➤ more than 20 nanaomoles/L are required to exclude androgen deficiency.

When a diagnosis of hypogonadism has been established, the underlying aetiology may also require investigation, particularly in the presence of secondary or hypogonadotrophic hypogonadism.

Treatment

Treatment is the same as for the general population, and should be considered. Treatment involves replacing the testosterone – transdermally, by intramuscular injection or with subdermally implanted pellets. Oral preparations are available but because of their relative inefficacy they provide a lower dose.

When patients do not adhere to treatment, signs of androgen deficiency persist and long-term complications are likely to occur.

Behavioural problems caused by testosterone therapy in patients with intellectual disability are not very common; behaviour sometimes improves.

DELAYED PUBERTY

When puberty fails to occur in a child with intellectual disability, it is frequently not regarded as a problem. However, there are major consequences of failure in pubertal development, including lack of appropriate growth and development, and the normal 'ageing process'. The decision of whether to treat the failure of normal pubertal development needs to be actively made, rather than allowing pubertal non-development, by default.

Testosterone should not be used in young boys without first consulting a paediatric endocrinologist.

CRYPTOORCHIDISM

Cryptoorchidism (undescended testes or testes not in the scrotum) is more common in hypogonadal males than in males with normal gonadal development.

Inguinal cryptoorchidism carries a four-fold, lifetime increased risk of testicular cancer; this risk is higher for an intra-abdominal testis. The risk is further increased in certain chromosomal disorders (possibly including Down syndrome). Inguinal testes are difficult to examine; there is justification for operating to bring them into the scrotum. In adults, intra-abdominal testes should be removed or at the very least should be brought into the scrotum to allow for routine regular surveillance.

Testicular surveillance

Testicular examination is recommended as self-care for young men. In men with intellectual disability, routine medical examination should include testicular palpation, especially of testes not in the scrotum (i.e. inguinal). Men with intellectual disability will not present if they feel a lump; support persons need to be aware of this.

In clinical practice, if one (or two) testes cannot be identified, a search for the undescended testis should be undertaken. Ultrasound examination is the first procedure in most patients.

INGUINAL HERNIA

Inguinal hernias found on routine examination do not always require treatment. Small asymptomatic direct inguinal hernias that are easily reducible can usually be observed. Any other hernias (and femoral hernias) should be considered for surgery.

Surgery is commonly performed under local anaesthetic; however, people with intellectual disability probably require a general anaesthetic, rather than concomitant sedation. The risks of general anaesthesia need to be weighed against the benefits of surgery. Surgery can be a day procedure, if appropriate postoperative analgesia is provided.

PROSTATE CANCER

Prostate cancer is common. A man has a lifetime risk of 16% (1 in 6) of being diagnosed with prostate cancer, and a 3% (1 in 33) chance of dying from it. The risk increases with age and is approximately 1 in 120 at age 55 years. Prostate cancer is more likely in men with a family history (a father or a brother) of prostate cancer, and in some ethnic groups. It is less common in men of Asian or Pacific Islander origin.

Symptoms

Prostate cancer is often asymptomatic. However, symptoms include blood in the urine, the need to urinate frequently (especially at night), weak or poor urine flow, pain or a burning feeling while urinating, an inability to urinate and constant pain in the back, pelvis or upper thighs.

Men with these symptoms require investigation. The symptoms can be attributed to many other causes including an enlarged prostate (very common) and infection.

Screening

Screening involves performing a test to separate an asymptomatic population into high-risk groups (requiring further investigation) and low-risk groups. Screening tests for prostate cancer include digital rectal examination and a 'prostate specific antigen' (PSA) blood test. Those who recommend screening encourage both tests.

There may be difficulty with the digital examination or it may cause misunderstanding in men with intellectual disability whose ability to communicate or understand concepts are limited.

The PSA blood test can be normal in men with prostate cancer and, conversely, not all high results mean cancer. About 15% of men over the age of 50 years have a higher than normal PSA; and of these only 1 in 5 (3%) will have prostate cancer.

Medical experts do not agree on the need for screening. The US Preventative Services Task Force concludes that there is not enough evidence to recommend screening at the present time. On the other hand, some experts recommend screening for men over the age of 50 years who have a further life expectancy of at least 10 years, particularly if they are in a high risk group (which includes men of African descent, or men with a father or brother who have had prostate cancer). Generally, it is recommended that information is given to individual men and, after appropriate counselling, for them to make an informed decision about whether to be screened. The decision of people with intellectual disability will involve others. There is a case for not screening most (if not all) men with intellectual disability, unless they have particularly strong risk factors.

ERECTILE DYSFUNCTION

Erectile dysfunction is common, with the prevalence increasing after the age of 40 years; by the age of 65 years between 25% and 45% of men have clinically significant erectile difficulties. The prevalence is possibly higher in men with intellectual disability because of the associated comorbidities. Associated medical conditions (including diabetes, neuropathy, vascular disease and hyperprolactinaemia) should be excluded.

Occasionally, a male with mild intellectual disability will complain of erectile dysfunction. The situation can be difficult for both the person with the disability and his support persons. Parents and other support persons often have preconceived ideas (often negative) about sexuality in people with intellectual disability. A man with intellectual disability who complains of erectile dysfunction should receive the same respect and treatment as would a man who does not have intellectual disability. For more information, *see also* Chapter 20, 'Sexuality' (p. 163).

EJACULATORY FAILURE

Ejaculatory failure is usually associated with autonomic neuropathy that is often seen after prostate or bowel surgery, or with diabetes. It does not require treatment unless fertility is an issue.

FURTHER READING

- Center J, Beange H, McElduff A. People with mental retardation have an increased prevalence of osteoporosis: a population study. *Am J Ment Retard.* 1998; **103**(1): 19–28.
- Conway AJ, Handelsman DJ, Lording DW, *et al.* Use, misuse and abuse of androgens. The Endocrine Society of Australia consensus guidelines for androgen prescribing. *Med J Aust.* 2000; **172**(5): 220–4.
- Harris R, Lohr KN. Screening for prostate cancer: an update of the evidence for the U.S. Preventive Services Task Force. *Ann Intern Med.* 2002; **137**(11): 917–29.
- McElduff A, Beange H. Men's health and wellbeing: testosterone deficiency. *J Intellect Dev Disabil.* 2003; **28**: 211–13.
- McElduff A, Center J, Beange H. Hypogonadism in men with intellectual disabilities: a population study. *J Intellect Dev Disabil.* 2003; **28**: 163–70.

CHAPTER 23

Legal issues: the Mental Capacity Act 2005

DECISION MAKING FOR ADULTS WITH IMPAIRED CAPACITY

In England and Wales the rights of adults with intellectual disability to make decisions about their care and future are enshrined in the Mental Capacity Act 2005 (MCA). In Scotland the Adults with Incapacity (Scotland) Act 2000 covers the same issues and in Northern Ireland there are no statutory provisions.

CAN THE PERSON MAKE THEIR OWN DECISION?

As a general rule all adults are presumed to be capable of making their own decisions, i.e. there is a presumption of capacity. Every adult has the right to make their own decisions if they have the capacity to do so. Some adults, however, have limited or no ability to make some or all decisions about their healthcare. The Mental Capacity Act is intended to be enabling and supportive of those who lack capacity, its purpose being to protect those who lack the capacity to make specific decisions, but also to maximise their ability to make decisions or to be part of the decision-making process.

The guiding statutory principles are enshrined in section 1 of the Mental Capacity Act 2005, which provides as follows.

➤ A person must be assumed to have capacity unless it is established that he lacks capacity.
➤ A person is not to be treated as unable to make a decision unless all practicable steps to help him to do so have been taken without success.
➤ A person is not to be treated as unable to make a decision merely because he makes an unwise decision.
➤ An act done, or decision made, under this Act for or on behalf of a person who lacks capacity must be done, or made, in his best interests.
➤ Before the act is done, or the decision is made, regard must be had to whether the purpose for which it is needed can be as effectively achieved in a way that is less restrictive of the person's rights and freedom of action.

These principles form the bedrock of the legislation. Before a conclusion is reached that an individual lacks capacity to make a particular decision it is vital that all possible steps are taken to try to help them reach a decision themselves.

Any act done for or any decision made on behalf of a person who lacks capacity must be in their 'best interests'.

Health professionals need to assess each situation and consider whether the person is capable of making a meaningful decision. It is important to balance a person's right to make a decision with their right to safety and protection when they cannot make decisions to protect themselves.

HELPING PEOPLE TO MAKE THE DECISION

Before deciding that someone lacks capacity to make a particular decision it is important to take all practical and appropriate steps to enable them to make that decision themselves.

There are numerous ways in which people can be helped and supported to make a decision for themselves:
➤ providing them with all of the relevant information to make a particular decision using, e.g. www.easyhealth.org
➤ ensuring that the information is provided in a comprehensible way, e.g. by using visual aids or simple language, or by the information being conveyed by a third party (e.g. a family member)
➤ making the person feel at ease, e.g. is there a particular location, like their home, where the person may feel more at ease in making any decision?

It might be necessary for the person to have access to advice from elsewhere, e.g. a family member, carer, trusted friend or a legal representative.

It is vital that good communication is used in explaining relevant and important information in an appropriate manner and for ensuring that steps are being taken to meet a person's needs (*see* Chapters 4 and 5).

Of course there might be emergency medical situations (e.g. if a person is unconscious) when urgent decisions have to be taken in a person's best interests. In such situations it may not be practical or indeed appropriate to delay treatment, but medical professionals must still try to communicate with the person and keep them informed of what is happening and what actions are being taken.

DEFINING MENTAL CAPACITY

Mental capacity is the ability to make a decision. The status of a person (e.g. being elderly), the outcome of a decision viewed by others as illogical, or the appearance or behaviour of a person may cause capacity to be questioned. However, outward appearances can create false impressions and it is therefore imperative that a proper assessment is undertaken using appropriate criteria. Therefore anyone assessing someone's capacity to make a decision for themselves should use the two-stage test identified in the MCA.

Stage 1 is to be found in section 2(1) MCA 2005 which provides:

> For the purposes of this Act, a person lacks capacity in relation to a matter if at the material time he is unable to make a decision for himself in relation to the matter because of an impairment of, or a disturbance in the functioning of, the mind or brain.

Stage 2 (the 'inability to make decisions') is to be found in section 3(1) MCA 2005:

For the purposes of section 2, a person is unable to make a decision for himself if he is unable –

- to understand the information relevant to the decision,
- to retain that information,
- to use or weigh that information as part of the process of making the decision, or
- to communicate his decision (whether by talking, using sign language or any other means).

The starting assumption must be that a person has the capacity to make a decision, unless it can be established that they lack capacity. A person's capacity must be assessed specifically in terms of their capacity to make a particular decision at the time it needs to be made and not their ability to make decisions in general.

Statutory safeguards are put in place (section 2(3) MCA) when a person's capacity is assessed since the decision must never be based simply on their age, appearance, or assumptions about their condition or any aspect of their behaviour.

In summary, a patient's capacity can be expressed in terms of the capacity to:
➤ receive, comprehend, retain and recall relevant information
➤ integrate the information received and relate it to the situation at hand
➤ evaluate benefits and risks in terms of personal values
➤ select an option and give convincing reasons for the choice
➤ be able to communicate the choice to others
➤ persevere with that choice (at least until the decision is acted upon).

Anyone who claims that a person lacks capacity must be able to provide proof and be able to establish, on a balance of probabilities, that the person lacks capacity to make a particular decision at the time it needs to be made, i.e. the person must be able to show that it is more likely than not that the person lacks capacity to make the decision in question.

Assessing capacity correctly is vitally important since someone who is assessed as lacking capacity may be denied their right to make a specific and fundamental decision. It is also important that those who undertake the assessment can justify their conclusions.

If a healthcare professional proposes an examination or treatment, they must assess the person's capacity to consent. In a hospital setting this might involve the decision being made by a multidisciplinary team, but ultimately it is up to the professional responsible for the person's treatment, often the GP, to make sure that capacity has been assessed.

Anyone assessing the person's capacity must not simply assume that a person lacks capacity because they have a particular diagnosis or medical condition. There must be proof that the diagnosed condition affects the person's ability to make a decision when it needs to be made. It is good practice for any such decisions to be recorded in the patient's clinical notes.

It must be remembered that no one can be forced to undergo an assessment of capacity. Clearly, if there are serious concerns about a person's mental health, an assessment under mental health legislation may be necessary (provided the statutory criteria are met).

BEST INTEREST DECISIONS

One of the key principles is that any act done for, or any decision made on behalf of, a person who lacks capacity must be done, or made, in that person's 'best interests'. Once it is established that a person lacks capacity there is a statutory checklist of factors which must be considered in deciding what is in a person's 'best interests'. Section 4 MCA provides as follows.

- In determining for the purposes of this Act what is in a person's best interests, the person making the determination must not make it merely on the basis of –
  (a) the person's age or appearance, or
  (b) a condition of his, or an aspect of his behaviour, which might lead others to make unjustified assumptions about what might be in his best interests.
- The person making the determination must consider all the relevant circumstances and, in particular, take the following steps.
- He must consider –
  (a) whether it is likely that the person will at some time have capacity in relation to the matter in question, and
  (b) if it appears likely that he will, when that is likely to be.
- He must, so far as reasonably practicable, permit and encourage the person to participate, or to improve his ability to participate, as fully as possible in any act done for him and any decision affecting him.
- Where the determination relates to life-sustaining treatment he must not, in considering whether the treatment is in the best interests of the person concerned, be motivated by a desire to bring about his death.
- He must consider, so far as is reasonably ascertainable –
  (a) the person's past and present wishes and feelings (and, in particular, any relevant written statement made by him when he had capacity),
  (b) the beliefs and values that would be likely to influence his decision if he had capacity, and
  (c) the other factors that he would be likely to consider if he were able to do so.
- He must take into account, if it is practicable and appropriate to consult them, the views of –
  (a) anyone named by the person as someone to be consulted on the matter in question or on matters of that kind,
  (b) anyone engaged in caring for the person or interested in his welfare,
  (c) any donee of a lasting power of attorney granted by the person, and
  (d) any deputy appointed for the person by the court,

  as to what would be in the person's best interests and, in particular, as to the matters mentioned in subsection (6).

SUSTAINING LIFE AND DNR NOTICES

Section 4(5) is worthy of comment in relation to the issue of sustaining life. Clearly, any decision about life sustaining treatment for a person lacking capacity will start from the assumption that it is in the person's best interests for life to continue. However, there will be some instances where it may be in the best interests of a patient to withdraw treatment or give palliative care (e.g. in the final stages of a terminal illness) that might incidentally shorten life. All of the best interest factors must be considered in such circumstances, including not being 'motivated by a desire to bring about his death'.

A particularly important element of the checklist is consideration being given to the person's 'wishes and feelings'. This clearly places the focus firmly on the person lacking capacity. However, their views will not automatically determine any outcome.

The statute also provides for family members, carers and other relevant people to be consulted on decisions affecting the person where 'practicable and appropriate'.

Provided acts or decisions as to care and treatment are in the 'best interests' of the person who lacks capacity, the decision maker or carer will be protected from liability.

The 'best interests' principles do not apply where someone has previously made an advance decision to refuse medical treatment while they had the capacity to do so and, in certain circumstances, persons lacking in capacity involved in research.

ACTS IN CONNECTION WITH CARE OR TREATMENT: 'THE PRINCIPLE OF NECESSITY'

Until the MCA, legislation had been silent about what actions could lawfully be taken by carers and healthcare professionals in looking after persons who lack capacity. In the absence of any statutory provision it was left to the Courts to establish the common law 'principle of necessity', setting out what actions and decisions could lawfully be taken. Section 5 MCA now makes statutory provision enabling carers and healthcare professionals to carry out certain tasks without fear of liability. The statute provides as follows in relation to care or treatment.

- If a person ('D') does an act in connection with the care or treatment of another person ('P'), the act is one to which this section applies if –
  (a) before doing the act, D takes reasonable steps to establish whether P lacks capacity in relation to the matter in question, and
  (b) when doing the act, D reasonably believes –
    i   that P lacks capacity in relation to the matter, and
    ii that it will be in P's best interests for the act to be done.
- D does not incur any liability in relation to the act that he would not have incurred if P –
  (a) had had capacity to consent in relation to the matter, and
  (b) had consented to D's doing the act.
- Nothing in this section excludes a person's civil liability for loss or damage, or his criminal liability, resulting from his negligence in doing the act.
- Nothing in this section affects the operation of sections 24 to 26 (advance decisions to refuse treatment).

The provisions are clearly intended to give legal backing for actions which are essential for the personal welfare/health of people lacking capacity to consent to having things done for them. The Code of Practice identifies a non-exhaustive list of actions covered by section 5 in relation to both what it terms 'personal care' and 'healthcare and treatment'. The list in relation to healthcare and treatment provides as follows:

➤ carrying out diagnostic examinations and tests (to identify an illness, condition or other problem)
➤ providing professional medical, dental and similar treatment
➤ giving medication
➤ taking someone to hospital for assessment or treatment
➤ providing nursing care (whether in hospital or in the community)
➤ carrying out any other necessary medical procedures (e.g. taking a blood sample) or therapies (e.g. physiotherapy or chiropody)
➤ providing care in an emergency.

Even if a person who lacks capacity to consent objects to the proposed treatment or admission to hospital the action might still be permissible under section 5 MCA. But it is important to emphasise that the actions in question will only receive protection from liability if the person is reasonably believed to lack capacity to give permission.

LIMITATIONS

There are limitations on acts which can be carried out with protection from liability relating to whether force or restraint can be used to impose treatment. These are to be found in section 6 MCA which provides as follows.

- If D does an act that is intended to restrain P, it is not an act to which section 5 applies unless two further conditions are satisfied.
- The first condition is that D reasonably believes that it is necessary to do the act in order to prevent harm to P.
- The second is that the act is a proportionate response to –
  (a) the likelihood of P's suffering harm, and
  (b) the seriousness of that harm . . .

Healthcare staff will clearly need to give careful consideration to these issues in relation to major healthcare and treatment decisions. Unless the person has previously made a lasting power of attorney (LPA) appoint someone to make such healthcare decisions for them or there is in existence a valid and applicable advance decision to refuse specific treatment, healthcare professionals will need to carefully consider what would be in a person's 'best interests'. The factors to consider are highlighted in section 5 MCA above.

LASTING POWER OF ATTORNEY

There are some situations where a person will want to provide another person authority to make a decision on their behalf. A power of attorney is a legal document that allows them to do so and an LPA is a form of a power of attorney created by the MCA.

Section 9 MCA provides as follows.

> A lasting power of attorney is a power of attorney under which the donor
> ('P') confers on the donee (or donees) authority to make decisions about
> all or any of the following –
>> (a) P's personal welfare or specified matters concerning P's personal
>> welfare, and
>> (b) P's property and affairs or specified matters concerning P's prop-
>> erty and affairs,
>
> and which includes authority to make such decisions in circumstances
> where P no longer has capacity.

As with all other aspects of the MCA, the presumption is that the person has capacity. It is only if it can be established that the person lacks capacity that the LPA is
triggered. By virtue of the LPA being able to make 'personal welfare' decisions this
will include healthcare and medical treatment issues, e.g. where a person should
live and decisions as to consenting/refusing medical examination and treatment.

The scope of the LPA's authority is extensive. In effect the attorney stands in the
place of the person lacking capacity and they can do whatever that person could do
for himself. There are, however, certain limitations that it is necessary to be aware
of, as follows.

➤ An LPA must be registered with the Office of the Public Guardian (OPG)
before it can be used. An unregistered LPA will not allow the attorney to
acquire any legal decision-making powers.
➤ The attorney's powers to make a decision might be restricted by the terms
of the instrument that originally established the LPA, e.g. an attorney can
only consent to or refuse life-sustaining treatment on behalf of the person
if the person has specifically stated in the LPA document that they want the
attorney to have this authority.
➤ Any decisions made by the attorney are made in the person's best interests as
identified in the MCA's core principles.

Ultimately the Court of Protection can intervene in relation to the operation of the
power and has the ability to cancel the LPA made in favour of the attorney, attach
conditions to the power, or extend the attorney's power beyond the scope of the
original document establishing the LPA.

ADVANCE DECISIONS CONCERNING REFUSAL OF TREATMENT

It is a general principle of law and medical practice that a competent adult has the
right to consent to or refuse medical treatment. The MCA provides statutory recognition for an adult's advance decision to consent to or refuse specified treatment
when competent to do so, which will come into effect when the adult becomes
incompetent (i.e. lacks capacity).

Section 24(1) MCA provides as follows.

> 'Advance decision' means a decision made by a person ('P'), after he has
> reached 18 and when he has capacity to do so, that if –

(a) at a later date and in such circumstances as he may specify, a specified treatment is proposed to be carried out or continued by a person providing healthcare for him, and

(b) at that time he lacks capacity to consent to the carrying out or continuation of the treatment,

the specified treatment is not to be carried out or continued.

An advance decision must be valid and applicable to the circumstances of the treatment proposed. If these factors are present, the decision has the effect as if the person had made it and had the capacity to make it. Healthcare professionals must follow the decision. To go against such a decision could be deemed to be an assault and to be in contravention of the person's human rights.

Once healthcare professionals have determined that a person lacks capacity to accept or refuse treatment at the relevant time it is necessary to ascertain whether an advance decision is valid and applicable. Healthcare professionals will need to consider the following factors.

➤ Has the person done anything that is quite clearly inconsistent with their advance decision?

➤ Has the person withdrawn their decision?

➤ Has the person subsequently conferred the power to make that decision on an attorney under an LPA?

➤ Are there reasonable grounds for believing that the person would have changed their decision if they had known more about the current circumstances?

All staff involved with the treatment of the person, as well as family members, should be given the opportunity to express their views concerning such matters. Ultimately, it is the responsibility of the healthcare professional in charge of the person's care to determine whether there is a valid and applicable advance decision.

If there is a fundamental question over whether an advance agreement exists (e.g. there is professional disagreement over the validity of an advance decision), an application should be made to the Court of Protection for what is termed a declaration. While such a decision of the Court is being sought healthcare professionals treating the person are not prevented from providing life-sustaining treatment or undertaking any act reasonably necessary to prevent a serious deterioration in the person's condition.

If the Court ultimately determines that an advanced decision is valid and applicable, it does not have the power to overturn it.

It might be the case that there is no one available to consult about the person's 'best interests' or there is no one whom it is appropriate to consult. In such circumstances an Independent Mental Capacity Advocate (IMCA) must be appointed to represent and support the person.

INDEPENDENT MENTAL CAPACITY ADVOCATE SERVICE

The MCA established this service to help vulnerable people who lack the capacity to make important decisions about serious medical treatment and changes of accommodation and who have no family or friends that it would be appropriate to consult. Put quite simply, it provides an independent safeguard for those people who have no one to speak on their behalf.

Section 35(4) MCA provides the following guiding principle.

> . . . a person to whom a proposed act or decision relates should, so far as practicable, be represented and supported by a person who is independent of any person who will be responsible for the act or decision.

An IMCA must be instructed and consulted for people lacking capacity who have no one else to support them whenever the following issues need determination:
➤ An NHS body is proposing to provide serious medical treatment.
➤ An NHS body or local authority is proposing to arrange or change accommodation in hospital or a care home and the person will remain in hospital longer than 28 days or they will stay in a care home for more than eight weeks.

Examples of 'serious medical treatment' are: major surgery, sterilisation and pregnancy termination.

It is of note that the duty to instruct an IMCA need not be followed if medical treatment is required as a matter of urgency. Clearly, any treatment thereafter will require the instruction of an IMCA. Where emergency treatment is undertaken a clear explanation for so doing should be recorded in the person's clinical records.

The role of the IMCA is to support and represent the person who lacks capacity. In undertaking this role they will strive to establish what the person's wishes and feelings might be. By virtue of their role they have the right to view relevant healthcare, social services and care home records relevant to their investigation. The IMCA might meet professionals or carers involved in the treatment or care of the person lacking capacity. If an issue arises concerning medical treatment they might even seek a second medical opinion.

The observations of the IMCA must be taken into account as part of the decision-making process as to whether a proposed decision is in a person's best interests. It is ultimately the decision-maker's responsibility to decide whether a proposed course of action is in the person's best interests.

THE COURT OF PROTECTION
Issues might arise as to a person's capacity to make a decision or what is determined to be in their best interests, e.g. there might be disagreements between family members and healthcare professionals as to treatment options, or professional disagreement between those assessing the person as to whether they have or lack capacity to make certain decisions.

It is clearly in the person's best interests for matters to be resolved quickly. Furthermore, it is in the best interests of all those involved with the individual's treatment, as well as family members, for matters to be resolved amicably and without recourse to litigation.

In cases where there is a doubt or dispute about whether a particular section 5 MCA act is in the person's best interests and the matter cannot be resolved through negotiation or other forms of dispute resolution then the Court of Protection has ultimate jurisdiction to resolve the matter.

Section 45 MCA establishes the new Court of Protection. Any decisions made by the Court must always follow the guiding principles contained in section 1 MCA and any decision must be in the best interests of the person concerned.

From a welfare perspective the Court has powers to:

➤ determine whether a person has capacity to make a decision for themselves (the lack of capacity must specifically relate to the particular issue before the court)
➤ make declarations, decisions or orders on welfare matters affecting a person who lacks capacity to make such specific decisions
➤ determine whether an LPA is valid, cancel the LPA made in favour of an attorney, attach conditions to the power, or extend the attorney's power beyond the scope of the original document establishing the LPA
➤ appoint a deputy to make a specified decision for a person lacking capacity on their behalf.

FURTHER READING

- Mental Capacity Act 2005.
- Mental Capacity Act 2005: Code of Practice; TSO.
- Hoghton M, Chadwick S. Assessing patient capacity. Remember CURB BADLIP in the UK. *BMJ*. 2010; **340**: c2767.

Part Three

Specific disorders associated with intellectual disability

CHAPTER 24

Down syndrome

Down syndrome is the most common identifiable genetic cause of intellectual disability with an incidence of approximately 1 in 800 live births. It is more common in older mothers but, as the majority of babies are born to younger women, most mothers of babies with Down syndrome are aged in their twenties. Despite a growing trend for women to have children later in life, the annual rate of Down syndrome births in the West is fairly constant. This is due to advances in prenatal screening leading to the termination of many affected pregnancies.

Down syndrome is a cause of intellectual disability and has many related medical issues (such as hypothyroidism and congenital malformations). Despite this, most interactions between people with Down syndrome and their general practitioner (GP) are for everyday medical problems that are unrelated to the syndrome. A GP must, however, be aware of the specialist services available in the area should the need arise.

Individuals with Down syndrome express the full range of human personality traits and it is important that they not be stereotyped as 'happy eternal children'.

AETIOLOGY

Approximately 92% of cases of Down syndrome have trisomy 21 in all cell lines, with the remaining 8% being split fairly evenly between mosaic forms and translocated forms. The most common translocation leading to Down syndrome is from the 21st to the 14th chromosome.

In at least 95% of cases of trisomy 21, the extra chromosome is maternally derived; however, determining the parent of origin usually serves no useful purpose. The chance of a couple who have conceived one child with trisomy 21 having a further pregnancy with Down syndrome is 1%, except in the case of balanced parental translocation, in which case the chance of recurrence is much higher.

The phenotypic features and the health and other problems associated with Down syndrome are a product of the over-expression of the genes on chromosome 21.

MANAGEMENT
General

Medical conditions that occur more frequently in people with Down syndrome include:

➤ leukaemias – 10 to 30 times more common throughout childhood
➤ transient myelodysplasia
➤ macrocytosis – which has no clinical significance
➤ epilepsy
➤ hearing deficits
➤ visual problems
➤ hypothyroidism – it is quite common for people with Down syndrome to have elevated thyroid stimulating hormone (TSH) in the presence of normal thyroid hormone levels. Thyroid replacement should not be given on the basis of an increased TSH level alone. The presence of thyroid autoantibodies correlates with an increased chance of developing true hypothyroidism
➤ coeliac disease – which may cause constipation or a number of other gastrointestinal symptoms, and should be considered if there are gastrointestinal complaints or failure to thrive
➤ constipation – if it fails to respond to appropriate dietary interventions, investigation for Hirschsprung's disease is recommended
➤ upper respiratory tract infections – possibly due to relative underdevelopment of the mid-face, and poor immunity. A relative size deficiency in the child's airways may also contribute
➤ otitis media – serous otitis media is a very common problem in children one to five years of age, and can persist for many years.

Recommendations for general screenings
The following areas require regular monitoring throughout the life of a person with Down syndrome (frequency of monitoring may vary with age – refer to specific age category also):
➤ biochemical screening for hypothyroidism
➤ hearing tests (usually standard techniques are sufficient) and tympanometry (the appropriate frequency to perform these two tests varies with age – refer to specific age category)
➤ regular evaluation of the middle ear space, and cleaning if necessary. If, due to small canals, the eardrum cannot be seen, the child should be sent to a specialist for evaluation and determination of necessary follow-up
➤ ophthalmological examination (frequency varies with age – refer to specific age category)
➤ immunisation – with the usual doses of vaccines, at the usual intervals
➤ regular dental checks.

Usual health screening as for the general population (and appropriate for age and sex) should also continue (e.g. blood pressure monitoring, cholesterol screening, breast or testes examination, cervical cytology). The establishment of good diet and exercise habits are also very important.

Secondary school (12 to 18 years)
Preventive health screening should include a cardiac examination, with particular attention to valvular disease. Dermatological issues are common in adolescence, especially folliculitis.
　　Health screening of note in this age group (*see also* the sections on general

management, p. 195, and recommendations for general screenings, p. 196):
- ➤ six-monthly screening for visual and auditory impairments
- ➤ annual otoscopic examinations
- ➤ monitoring of oropharyngeal and nasopharyngeal lymphoid tissue growth (as overgrowth of lymphoid tissue can lead to sleep apnoea and cor pulmonale)
- ➤ six-monthly biochemical screening for hypothyroidism
- ➤ monitoring of weight to ensure weight gain is appropriate
- ➤ screen for coeliac disease.

Sexuality and fertility
WOMEN

Menarche occurs at the usual time in women with Down syndrome and the vast majority of young women will ovulate. Most women with Down syndrome can manage their menstruation either independently or with varying degrees of assistance. Pain and other premenstrual symptoms may cause an increase in difficult behaviour in women with Down syndrome. Education on appropriate sexual expression and protective behaviours, and reliable contraception, is important.

Women with Down syndrome have a higher than usual risk of medical complications in pregnancy, and should be referred to specialist services when they become pregnant.

For more information, *see* Chapter 7, 'The Adolescent with Intellectual Disability' (p. 47) and Chapter 21, 'Women's Health' (p. 169).

MEN

Males with Down syndrome undergo puberty at a similar age as males in the general population do. More than 25% of boys with Down syndrome have undescended testes. Males with Down syndrome are usually presumed to be infertile; however, the reason for their infertility is unknown. *See also* Chapter 7, 'The Adolescent with Intellectual Disability' (p. 47) and Chapter 22, 'Men's Health' (p. 178).

Obesity
Although people with Down syndrome appear to be predisposed to being overweight, appropriate food intake and activity levels can offset any gain in weight. As metabolic rate may be lower in those with Down syndrome, any dietary advice needs to take the decreased metabolic rate into account. Obesity predisposes people to obstructive sleep apnoea.

Obstructive sleep apnoea
Sleep apnoea, which is worsened by obesity, occurs more commonly than usual in children and adolescents with Down syndrome but the symptoms may be obscured by communication difficulties. Headache, irritability, somnolence and behavioural change may all be caused by sleep apnoea. Parents should be asked about snoring and breathing irregularities in their children at night, but as the parents' reporting is not always accurate a sleep study may be necessary.

Adulthood

Some adults with Down syndrome can live relatively independently; others require varying support from their families or external agencies. One option for accommodation is independent living with outreach support; however, the available places are generally less than the demand.

Employment may be available in a range of supported environments. However, although many individuals are capable of employment (with varying levels of support), it is not always available. Lack of adequate employment can lead to negative consequences for the individual and other family members. If a person with Down syndrome cannot be left at home alone, other family members may be obliged to give up employment to care for them.

Adults who are home alone for long periods of time may become very sedentary, watching inordinate amounts of television. The individual should be strongly encouraged to become involved in activities they find meaningful. Loneliness can be a significant issue.

Medical concerns

Early adulthood is the peak time for development of hypothyroidism; mitral valve prolapse may also occur at this age. The incidence of epilepsy begins to rise steadily through adult life, after an initial peak during infancy. Osteoporosis is more common in those with Down syndrome than in both the general population and people with intellectual disability from other causes. Sleep apnoea continues to be a risk factor and should be monitored.

Any person with a history of institutionalised care may have been exposed to *Helicobacter pylori* and a number of other infectious diseases (e.g. tuberculosis, hepatitis B) and should be screened.

Most adults with Down syndrome develop periodontal disease, which is a leading cause of tooth loss; their oral health should be checked regularly. *See also* Chapter 19, 'Oral Health', p. 160.

Women with Down syndrome appear to experience early onset menopause, with one study reporting a mean age of 44.6 years.

Health screening of note in this age group (*see also* the sections on general management, p. 195, and recommendations for general screenings, p. 196):

➤ annual thyroid function screening
➤ annual cardiovascular examination and (if clinical uncertainty exists) echocardiogram
➤ electroencephalogram (if clinically indicated).

Mental health concerns

Psychiatric illness is more commonly diagnosed in people with Down syndrome than in the general population. Individuals with Down syndrome may experience a range of psychiatric disturbances including mania, obsessive compulsive disorder, anorexia nervosa, Tourette syndrome, schizophrenia and phobia.

There is some evidence that adults with Down syndrome are particularly vulnerable to depression. Sensory deficits and medical illness (such as hypothyroidism and sleep apnoea) may account for some of the reported symptomatology. However, the individual's environment and personal circumstances also need consideration before a diagnosis is made. A trial of medication may be worthwhile as the response can be dramatic, and non-treatment of depression impairs the quality of life. If life circumstances are thought to be a contributing factor, referral to appropriate services should be undertaken.

Aged care

In 1960, the mean age of death for people with Down syndrome was 21 years. Life expectancy has increased significantly in the last 40 years, with the mean age of death now being in the sixth decade. Reasons for this include surgical correction of congenital abnormalities of the heart, improved nutrition and healthier living conditions.

Individuals with Down syndrome are at increased risk of age-related visual and hearing problems.

Dementia and Alzheimer's disease

Current theories about the metabolic impact of trisomy 21 suggest that overexpression of relevant genes on the 21st chromosome leads to early onset of age-related conditions such as Alzheimer's disease. There is evidence that Alzheimer's disease occurs up to two decades earlier in people with Down syndrome; however, the true incidence of the disease is difficult to establish as there appears to be a lack of synchrony between the neuropathology of the disease and changes in behaviour.

Work towards a formal diagnosis of dementia should only proceed after exclusion of these conditions and any detected pathologies have been treated.

A person with Down syndrome who is diagnosed with Alzheimer's disease should remain in their current accommodation and occupational settings (with appropriate modifications, as necessary) for as long as possible; the practitioner can become involved in efforts to facilitate this. Treatment with cholinesterase inhibitors is started after a full assessment.

ROLE OF THE GENERAL PRACTITIONER

Individuals should be given the opportunity to participate in their own healthcare to the extent that they are capable. Illness prevention (e.g. dietary and exercise management) is an area where the individual's involvement is important. Self-management of these, and other issues, is only possible if information has been provided regularly and in an appropriate form. GPs who have ongoing contact with a patient are in an ideal position to initiate and support the appropriate learning of healthy behaviours. *See also* Chapter 8, 'Adult Healthcare' (p. 56), Chapter 10, 'Preventive Healthcare and Health Promotion' (p. 80) and Chapter 9, 'Aged Care' (p. 67).

Practitioners can use any opportunity to talk about practical issues that may impact on the individual's well-being and development, such as family functioning, stress of family members, knowledge of available resources (such as respite care) and whether the individual has a loving and stimulating environment.

Other therapies

Practitioners are often asked about nutritional and physical therapies that have been promoted as being cures, or at least significantly efficacious in ameliorating the disability associated with Down syndrome. The common feature of all these therapies is their lack of evidence of efficacy. There is certainly not enough evidence to support their recommendation by medical practitioners. Rather than dismissing the carer's request for advice, however, practitioners can help individuals to make informed choices about the use of such therapies.

A number of parents choose alternative and/or complementary medicine for their child with Down syndrome. The GP should always ask if they are being given, so that this information can be considered when medical interventions are being discussed.

FURTHER READING

- Carr J. *Down's Syndrome: growing up.* Cambridge: Cambridge University Press; 1995.
- Collacott RA. Down syndrome and mental health needs. In: Bouras N, editor. *Psychiatric and Behavioural Disorders in Developmental Disabilities and Mental Retardation.* Cambridge: Cambridge University Press; 1999, pp. 200–11.
- Down Syndrome Medical Interest Group. Healthcare guidelines for individuals with Down syndrome: 1999 revision. *Down Syndrome Quarterly.* 1999; **4**(3): 1–16.
- Henderson A, Lynch SA, Wilkinson S, *et al.* Adults with Down's syndrome: the prevalence of complications and health care in the community. *Br J Gen Pract.* 2007; **57**: 50–5.
- Holland AJ, Hon J, Huppert FA, *et al.* Incidence and course of dementia in people with Down's syndrome: findings from a population-based study. *J Intellect Disabil Res.* 2000; **44**(2): 138–46.
- Mantry D, Cooper S-A, Smiley E, *et al.* The prevalence and incidence of mental ill-health in adults with Down syndrome. *J Disabil Res.* 2008; **52**(2): 141–55.
- Melville CA, Cooper S-A, McGrother CW, *et al.* Obesity in adults with Down syndrome: a case-control study. *J Intellect Disabil Res.* 2005; **49**(2): 125–33.
- Roizen NJ. Medical care and monitoring for the adolescent with Down syndrome. *Adolesc Med.* 2002; **13**(2): 345–58, vii.
- Zachor DA. Down syndrome and celiac disease: a review. *Down Syndrome Quarterly.* 2000; **5**(4): 1–5.
- Zigman WB, Lott IT. Alzheimer's disease in Down syndrome: neurobiology and risk. *Ment Retard Dev Disabil Res Rev.* 2007; **13**: 237–46.

CHAPTER 25

Cerebral palsy

Cerebral palsy is a persistent but not unchanging disorder of movement and posture due to a defect or lesion of the developing brain. The prevalence is about 2.0 to 2.5 per 1000 live births. The majority of children with cerebral palsy live to adulthood and so 'cerebral palsy must be regarded as a condition with which people live rather than a condition from which they die'. Individuals may begin to experience the effects of ageing in their early thirties. Clinical management of adults with cerebral palsy may be complicated by the person's inability to communicate with the doctor, resulting in an inaccurate or incomplete health history. Consequently, it is important to evaluate each person as an individual and to encourage patients and their support persons to maintain accurate health records.

AETIOLOGY

There are many different causes of cerebral palsy. There is a strong association with low birthweight and prematurity. In a considerable proportion of cases, the cause remains unknown.

It is important to establish the cause of cerebral palsy if possible. Information about the cause of the disability is helpful for families and essential for genetic counselling. Investigations such as urinary metabolic screening and chromosome analysis may elucidate rare causes of cerebral palsy. Radiological procedures such as MRI can be useful if preliminary investigations have been negative.

Prenatal events

Prenatal events are thought to be responsible for approximately 75% of all causes of cerebral palsy. Known causes include congenital intrauterine infection (e.g. rubella, cytomegalovirus, toxoplasmosis), vascular events (e.g. middle cerebral artery occlusion) and malformations (e.g. the cortical dysplasias).

Perinatal events

Perinatal asphyxia accounts for about 8% to 10% of all cases of cerebral palsy. Birth asphyxia may be caused by antepartum haemorrhage, or other placental or cord problems. Neonatal problems such as severe hypoglycaemia or untreated jaundice may be responsible for cerebral palsy in some individuals.

Postnatal events

Postnatal events account for about 10% of all cases. Known causes include:
➤ accidental injury (e.g. hypoxic events [such as near-drowning accidents], head trauma [such as from motor vehicle accidents])
➤ non-accidental injury or child abuse
➤ severe brain infections (e.g. meningitis).

CLASSIFICATION

Cerebral palsy may be classified in three ways:
1 Type of motor disorder (e.g. spasticity, dyskinesia, ataxia, mixed).
   a Spasticity – is the most common type of motor disorder and accounts for about 70% of all cases. Spasticity involves increased muscle tone with characteristic clasp-knife quality. Clinical features include impaired control of voluntary movement, clonus, hyperreflexia and weakness. Contractures often result.
   b Dyskinesia (athetosis or dystonia) – almost always affects the whole body (including all four limbs) and generally results from damage to the basal ganglia. It is characterised by variable muscle tone, dysarthria, loss of control of body posture and involuntary movements.
   c Ataxia – refers to a disorder of balance associated with damage to the cerebellum; unsteadiness, tremor and hypotonicity may be present.
   d Mixed – refers to a mixture of more than one type of cerebral palsy. This is common, particularly the combination of spasticity and athetosis.
2 Distribution of the motor disorder (e.g. hemiplegia, diplegia, quadriplegia).
3 Severity of the motor disorder, which in children is best described using the Gross Motor Function Measure (a five-level, ordinal grading system based on functional abilities) and the need for assistive technology and wheeled mobility.

PRESENTATION AND DIAGNOSIS

Adults with an established diagnosis of cerebral palsy may present for management of other acute or chronic health issues. A decrease in overall functioning may be related to the interaction between lifelong motor impairment, associated conditions, ageing and age-related disease.

MANAGEMENT

The management of adults with cerebral palsy involves:
➤ establishing appropriate communication techniques
➤ performing annual full physical, psychological and social assessment
➤ managing the disorders and health problems associated with cerebral palsy
➤ assessing and managing other presenting health issues
➤ referring to, and liaising with, allied health professionals; annual reassessment may be necessary in some individuals
➤ providing support and information for the individual, their family or other support persons.

Management of associated health problems

The major health problems associated with cerebral palsy and the recommendations for their management are listed below:

> ➤ hearing – two- to five-yearly review by an audiologist
> ➤ vision – two- to five-yearly review by an optometrist/ophthalmologist
> ➤ epilepsy – monitor antiepileptics regularly and be aware of adverse effects of medication
> ➤ nutrition – beware of obesity and undernutrition; involve dietician/speech pathologist; nasogastric or gastrostomy feeding may be indicated
> ➤ oral health – six-monthly dental check
> ➤ poor saliva control – involve speech pathologist, consider medication and surgery
> ➤ gastro-oesophageal disease – be aware of increased risk and unusual presentation (e.g. difficulty swallowing, aspiration, or anaemia from blood loss with oesophageal ulceration). Pain may be expressed non-verbally (e.g. screaming or behaviour change)
> ➤ genitourinary problems – assess reason for occurrence; check for undescended testes
> ➤ constipation – evaluate diet and fluid intake; use laxatives appropriately
> ➤ chronic lung disease – assess for eating and swallowing difficulties; recurrent chest problems may be a sign of aspiration; refer to speech pathologist if suspected
> ➤ musculoskeletal effects:
>   – ongoing management by physician, physiotherapist and orthopaedic surgeon to maintain range of movement, muscle strength, independent mobility and realistic levels of physical exercise, and to reduce muscle fatigue and pain
>   – manage scoliosis and kyphosis
>   – manage spasticity
> ➤ psychological health – be aware of the risk of psychiatric disorders and psychological impairment; address body image and sexuality issues
> ➤ other issues – communication difficulties, intellectual disability, perceptual problems, osteoporosis.

A more detailed discussion follows; *see also* further information in Chapter 8, 'Adult Healthcare' (p. 56).

Hearing

All adults with cerebral palsy need their hearing assessed every two to five years. Hearing problems occur frequently and may remain undetected.

Vision

Individuals with cerebral palsy have special eye care needs and they require a visual assessment every two to five years. Visual disorders, particularly strabismus, are common. Refractive errors can remain undetected.

Epilepsy

Epilepsy occurs in approximately 20% of adults with cerebral palsy. It is most common in those with severe motor problems and requires careful management. The aims of therapy are to minimise the number of seizures and so reduce morbidity and mortality and to optimise the individual's independence and participation in activities and thus improve their quality of life.

Regular review of antiepileptic medication is important. Drug serum level estimation is only useful for carbamazepine, phenytoin and phenobarbitone. Levels of these drugs should be checked if clinically indicated (e.g. uncontrolled seizures, possible adverse effects).

There is evidence that individuals who have been on antiepileptic medication (including the newer antiepileptics) for many years are at increased risk of osteoporosis and, therefore, fractures. Skeletal monitoring (densitometry) is therefore indicated in people on long-term antiepileptic therapy. Important osteoporosis-prevention strategies in this population include ensuring an adequate source of calcium and vitamin D, and encouraging weightbearing, where possible. *See also* Chapter 16, 'Epilepsy' (p. 137).

Nutrition

Nutritional problems, particularly obesity and undernutrition, are commonly seen. Obesity may be due to lack of regular physical activity and poor dietary habits causing exacerbation of arthritis and scoliosis, and difficulties with independent mobility. Poor oral hygiene, oropharyngeal uncoordination, gastro-oesophageal disease and dysphagia may contribute to problems with undernutrition. Nasogastric or gastrostomy feeds should be considered if there is failure to thrive, excessively long mealtimes, or aspiration. *See also* Chapter 17, 'Nutritional Disorders' (p. 146).

Education regarding good dietary habits is essential. Involving a dietician and speech pathologist often helps.

Oral health

Due to chewing and swallowing difficulties and common dental conditions such as overbite, people with cerebral palsy are particularly susceptible to dental problems. Malocclusions are prevalent because of abnormal muscle function. Dental health should be regularly monitored, with dental visits six-monthly if possible.

Periodontal disease leads to halitosis, dental caries and the early loss of teeth. Education should centre on correct oral hygiene techniques and dietary modification. Lack of education, and the inability of support persons to correctly brush and floss teeth, may complicate effective oral hygiene.

Sometimes dental procedures need to be carried out under general anaesthesia. Liaison between the GP and the dentist may be required to discuss the individual's medication regimen. *See also* Chapter 19, 'Oral Health' (p. 160).

Poor saliva control

The social implications of drooling are important. Referral to a speech pathologist is helpful in managing poor saliva control, and paediatricians, dentists, otolaryngologists and plastic surgeons may also have a role in the management of this problem. Management strategies may include:
- eating and drinking modification
- orofacial facilitation
- appliances such as myofunctional devices and palatal training devices – both are rarely used
- behavioural management
- deodorising agents for odour problems due to stale saliva

➤ anticholinergic medication (benzhexol and benztropine or hyoscine patches)
➤ surgery – may be indicated when conservative approaches have failed; dental health should be carefully monitored following saliva control surgery, as there is a slightly increased risk of dental caries.

Gastro-oesophageal disease

Gastro-oesophageal reflux, oesophagitis and oesophageal bleeding are all common problems in people with severe cerebral palsy. Upper gastrointestinal tract bleeding is a common cause of hospitalisation, particularly in patients who have a combination of spastic quadriplegia and intellectual disability. Chronic reflux oesophagitis is a significant cause of aspiration pneumonia.

Oesophagitis may be difficult to diagnose because the patient may not be able to report the symptoms, and those symptoms commonly seen in the general population are often not elicited in people with disability. People with gastro-oesophageal disease may present with non-specific deterioration in the level of functioning; anaemia from subclinical blood loss; anorexia, vomiting and/or frank upper gastrointestinal haemorrhage; pain and/or irritability; behavioural change; or halitosis. Complications of untreated reflux disease include ulceration, anaemia, stricture formation, Barrett's oesophagitis and aspiration pneumonia.

Appropriate investigations include a full blood count to assess the haemoglobin level. These patients often require referral to a gastroenterologist for gastroscopy and further assessment.

Management may include positioning the person appropriately during mealtimes (a speech therapist or occupational therapist may be able to suggest other helpful techniques), medication (acid suppressing agents), and antireflux surgery (e.g. Nissen fundoplication, gastrostomy).

Genitourinary problems

Urinary incontinence and retention are common problems for both men and women with cerebral palsy. Neurological dysfunction, urinary tract infection, infrequent voiding, inability or difficulty physically accessing the toilet, and sensory deficits, may all be contributing factors.

Physical assessment, including urological referral if necessary, should be the first step in dealing with urinary problems. Behaviour management and assessment of the environment may be of benefit; input from an occupational therapist and psychologist may help.

Undescended testes are a common but often unrecognised problem that, if not addressed, carries an associated cancer risk. Check for this condition when examining adult patients for the first time. Screening for other genital problems, for both men and women, should be in line with general population recommendations.

Constipation

Children and adults often develop constipation due to insufficient intake of dietary fibre and fluids, and a lack of regular physical activity.

Encourage individuals to follow the same routine, where possible, in attempting to achieve regular bowel habits. Educate the individual and their carers of the importance of dietary fibre, adequate fluid intake and physical activity in achieving regular bowel evacuation. Inform them that routines and the post-meal gastrocolic reflex are important in bowel management. If these strategies are ineffective, laxatives may help. *See also* the section on constipation, p. 59.

Chronic lung disease

Some individuals with severe cerebral palsy develop chronic lung disease due to aspiration from oromotor dysfunction or severe gastro-oesophageal reflux; aspiration may occur silently for some time. *See also* the section on gastro-oesophageal reflux disease (p. 58). The presence of coughing during mealtimes, or wheezing during or after meals, may draw attention to the possibility of aspiration. Aspiration may result in recurrent pneumonia. Respiratory conditions are the most significant cause of mortality in people with cerebral palsy.

Regular surveillance by the GP or medical specialist is recommended. If there is a suspicion of eating or swallowing problems, assessment by a speech pathologist is often helpful. There is no definitive test for aspiration, but barium videofluoroscopy may help to clarify the situation. In the presence of aspiration, alternative feeding regimens such as the use of gastrostomy should be considered. *See also* the section on enteral tube feeding (p. 149).

Musculoskeletal effects

The physiotherapist plays a central role in the management of individuals with cerebral palsy.

Ongoing physiotherapy for adults may help maintain physical independence and movement, and may reduce muscle fatigue and pain. In people with cerebral palsy, abnormal stress and strain on joints and limbs often leads to early onset of conditions related to wear and tear (e.g. arthritis).

Immobilising a limb of a person with cerebral palsy is often difficult, and more vigorous treatment regimens than usual (including ultrasound and joint injection) may be required.

LOWER LIMB

Early detection of developmental dysplasia of the hip is important but if it has been missed expert orthopaedic assessment of the patient in adulthood is needed.

Flexion contractures at the knee may require hamstring surgery.

Equinus deformity at the ankle is the most common orthopaedic problem in children with cerebral palsy, and again may need expert orthopaedic or podiatric management in adulthood.

Gait analysis may assist in the planning and evaluation of orthopaedic surgical procedures.

UPPER LIMB

Shoulder dislocations and subluxations may occur in adults, and require treatment. Referral for physiotherapy and occupational therapy is recommended.

Surgical procedures to improve and maintain function of the hands (e.g. tenotomies and tendon transplants) require careful assessment.

SCOLIOSIS

Scoliosis develops in adolescence, and may lead to increased respiratory problems, decreased mobility, and increased joint and muscle pain. Attention to seating (including special seating aids) for those with postural changes associated with muscle contractures is required. Management may also include surgical intervention such as spinal fusion (especially in adolescence).

SPASTICITY

Management of spasticity can improve function and comfort. It requires a team approach. Focal spasticity can be treated by injection of botulinum toxin type A or the use of nerve blocks.

For generalised spasticity, oral medications are most commonly used to facilitate care or to inhibit painful muscle spasms. The most commonly used medications are diazepam, dantrolene and baclofen.

➤ Diazepam is a good antispasticity agent but may result in adverse effects (particularly drowsiness) if given in doses that are adequate to reduce muscle tone.

➤ Dantrolene is often ineffective and can cause hepatotoxicity.

➤ Baclofen can cause sedation, and does not cross the blood–brain barrier well. However, if given intrathecally by means of a pump implanted under the skin, it is much more effective than oral therapy. Intrathecal baclofen is only suitable for a small number of patients with severe spasticity. The risk of adverse reactions, the cost of the pump, the necessity for frequent medical appointments for pump refills and the need for pump replacement after about seven years must all be thoroughly considered by the patient, their family and the treating team before initiating treatment. The goals should be carefully established. The ultimate goal in using this technology is often to improve quality of life.

Another treatment option is selective dorsal rhizotomy where anterior spinal roots are sectioned to reduce spasticity; this is an irreversible procedure and appropriate patient selection is critical to a good outcome.

Specialists in rehabilitation medicine can provide useful advice about the treatment options.

Psychological health

Psychological impairments in people with cerebral palsy are common and can be easily overlooked or remain untreated. They may be responsible for suboptimal performance either with academic tasks or with self-care. Adolescents and adults with cerebral palsy commonly experience depression, frustration, anxiety and anger. Communication impairments, limited independence, changes in functional ability and barriers to social access may contribute to these feelings. Medication interactions can also lead to behavioural changes or other problems.

Review of current life circumstances, relationships, opportunities and supports may be of benefit. Referral to a psychologist and/or psychiatrist may also be helpful.

Communication difficulties

Common communication difficulties include dysarthria, hearing and vision impairments and cognitive deficits. Communication can be further impeded by fatigue, sedation (due to medications or alcohol) and medical conditions. Difficulties with communication may lead to frustration and misdiagnosis of illnesses.

Many people with cerebral palsy use augmentative communication techniques such as symbols, communication boards and electronic devices. Carers may also assist in the communication process. Because of the communication difficulties, extra time is often required in a consultation so that correct information exchange can occur. *See also* Chapter 5, 'Methods of Communication' (p. 34).

Intellectual disability

Approximately 40% to 45% of people with cerebral palsy have levels of functioning in the mild intellectual disability range or below. This does not necessarily correlate with the severity of the physical disability. Children and adults may benefit from formal cognitive assessment and may need ongoing help with their educational, vocational or occupational programmes.

Perceptual problems

Perceptual problems occur frequently. Motor planning difficulties, eye–hand coordination and problems of spatial awareness and shape recognition can impact on the person's organisational abilities and living skills. An occupational therapist and educational psychologist can provide assessment and advice.

HEALTH ISSUES RELATED TO AGEING

Adults with cerebral palsy commonly suffer from conditions associated with the normal process of ageing as early as in their twenties and thirties (e.g. unexpected fatigue, loss of physical function and independence, increased frustration).

These are treatable conditions of ageing and should not be considered as unchangeable characteristics of cerebral palsy. Practitioners should encourage patients to access appropriate community resources, such as leisure activities and home supports, when required.

REFERRALS

An adult with cerebral palsy may require referral to allied health professionals on either a regular or an 'as required' basis.

➤ Physiotherapists provide advice and training about methods to encourage movement, and information about orthotics, walking aids and special seating.
➤ Occupational therapists aid the development of self-care and upper-limb skills, and provide advice about equipment and home modifications.
➤ Speech therapists assist in the development of speech and communication, and provide guidance about feeding difficulties and saliva control problems. They also advise on the use and availability of augmentative communication devices.
➤ Psychologists provide functional assessment of adults, vocational aptitude testing, skills training and management of challenging behaviours.
➤ Other useful referrals include nurses, dieticians, social workers, orthotists, orthoptists, ophthalmologists and other medical specialists.

FURTHER READING

- Graham HK, Selber P. Musculoskeletal aspects of cerebral palsy. *J Bone Joint Surg (Br)*. 2002; **85**(B): 157–66.

- Hemmings K, Hutton JL, Pharoah POD. Long-term survival for a cohort of adults with cerebral palsy. *Dev Med Child Neurol.* 2006; **48**: 90–5.
- Rosenbaum P. Cerebral palsy: what parents and doctors want to know. *BMJ.* 2003; **326**: 970–4.
- Stanley FJ, Blair E, Alberman E. *Cerebral Palsies: epidemiology and causal pathways. Clinics in developmental medicine.* London: MacKeith Press; 2000.
- Tracy JM, Wallace R. Presentations of physical illness in people with developmental disability: the example of gastro-oesophageal reflux. *Med J Aust.* 2001; **175**(2): 109–11.

CHAPTER 26

Autism spectrum conditions

DEFINITIONS

Autism spectrum conditions (ASC), autistic spectrum disorder (ASD) or autism are all terms used to describe a group of lifelong neurodevelopment conditions with onset usually before the age of three years. This group of disorders is 'characterised' by a triad of behavioural issues as follows.

1 Impairment of social interaction and development

The reduced social skills, such as being unable to apparently share emotions, or reduced understanding of how others think and feel (lack of empathy), may severely restrict interactions with others. Children with ASC are less likely to take turns and may attempt non-verbal communication, such as leading another person's hand. Some may have tantrums and aggressive challenging behaviour which can lead to further social isolation.

2 Impairment of verbal and non-verbal communication

A significant proportion of individuals with ASC do not develop enough speech to meet their daily communication needs. Eye contact, smiling and responding to social stimuli are generally reduced. This may lead the person to be cut off, but they may be able to recognise and engage emotionally when their body language is mirrored to them, as is used in the communication technique of intensive interaction.

3 Repetitive behaviours

People with ASC may have routines or repetitive behaviours, e.g.

➤ repeating words or actions over and over (stereotypy)
➤ obsessively following routines or schedules (ritualistic behaviour)
➤ playing with toys or objects in repetitive and sometimes inappropriate ways
➤ having very specific and inflexible ways of arranging items (sameness and compulsive behaviour).

Thirty per cent of children with ASC will have self-injury behaviour at some stage. All these behaviours may occur with other conditions but appear to be more severe and frequent in ASC.

As clinicians we may use the terms autism, autistic spectrum disorder and pervasive development disorder (PDD) interchangeably, but this terminology can be confusing for others including parents, carers and teachers. The term autistic spectrum conditions (ASC) is less pejorative than others and is increasingly used as the favoured diagnostic terminology.

Without the expertise of parents and teachers, however, few of us can really gain any insight into what it must feel like to have an autistic spectrum condition or to live with someone who does.

A person with ASC may be affected in a broad spectrum of manifestations, including severely affected individuals (who may be apparently socially unresponsive, intellectually disabled and locked into repetitive movements such as hand flapping, rocking or apparent self-harming behaviour) to high-functioning individuals (who may be functioning 'normally' in society but may have narrowly focused interests, distinctly unusual social approaches, and pedantic communication).

THE THREE MAIN ASC GROUPS
Autistic spectrum conditions contain three main groups as follows.

1 'Classic' autism or autistic disorder
People with autism usually have significant language delays, social and communication challenges, and unusual behaviours and interests. All levels of IQ can occur in association with autism, but there are significant levels of intellectual disability in 75% of people with ASD.

2 Asperger syndrome
People with Asperger syndrome may appear to have milder symptoms of autistic disorder as they typically do not have problems with language or intellectual disability. They usually have qualitative impairment in social interactions with social challenges and unusual behaviours and interests. Typically, their conversations are characterised by a narrow subject with one-sided verbosity and restricted variation in rhythm and intonation of their speech.

Physical clumsiness and lack of empathy are typical of the condition. Unlike most people with ASC, people with Asperger syndrome are not usually withdrawn but it is their lack of empathy and reciprocity that interferes with developing friendships and they may appear socially awkward.

3 Pervasive developmental disorder – not otherwise specified (PDD-NOS)
This is also referred to as atypical personality development, atypical PDD or atypical autism.

People who meet some of the criteria for autistic disorder or Asperger syndrome, but not all, may be diagnosed with PDD-NOS. People with PDD-NOS usually have fewer and milder symptoms than those with autistic disorder. However, there are still marked impairments of social interaction and communication and should not be seen as a slightly autistic.

Rett syndrome
Rett syndrome (*see* Chapter 30) has distinct characteristics and diagnostic criteria.

PREVALENCE

The prevalence of autistic spectrum conditions in school children in the UK is estimated at 1%. This is similar to the prevalence in the US of 1 in 110 children in 2006. In 2009 the UK government passed the Autism Bill which allows local authorities in England and Wales to record the number of children with autism. Assuming the average list size of a whole time equivalent, a GP can expect to be involved in the care of up to 20 people with ASC.

DIAGNOSIS AND SCREENING

In the UK parents usually present children for a diagnosis to their health visitor or GP after concerns about development or behaviour, in contrast to the US and Japan where infants are screened at 18 months for ASC. The GP should be alerted to these possible red flag indicators for ASC:

➤ does not babble, point or make meaningful gestures by one year
➤ does not speak single words by 16 months
➤ does not combine two words by two years other than echolalia
➤ does not respond to name
➤ loses language or social skills at any age.

The GP or health visitor could use the Checklist for Autism in Toddlers (CHAT) at 18 months to screen children (*see* www.autism.org.uk/Working-with/Health/Screening-and-diagnosis/Checklist-for-autism-in-toddlers-CHAT.aspx). If the child fails, the test is repeated in four weeks, and the child is referred to a specialist paediatric service if there are concerns. The paediatrician may use several standard diagnostic instruments and tools. The diagnosis is based on behaviour and is defined in the DSM-IV-TR and ICD-10 as exhibiting at least six symptoms in total, including at least two symptoms of qualitative impairment in social interaction, at least one symptom of qualitative impairment in communication, and at least one symptom of restricted and repetitive behaviour.

Early diagnosis is important both for the child and the family. Early invention for the child and obtaining a statement of special educational needs allows access to specialist health services and improves outcomes for the child. The diagnosis helps families to plan their care and domestic arrangements and consider whether to have further children after genetic testing, particularly for fragile X syndrome. In the UK the National Autism Plan for Children recommends at most 30 weeks from first concern to diagnosis, but this is seldom the case and considerable numbers of children and families have to wait until after the child is five years old. The delay in diagnosis causes considerable distress to families and prevents potential early intervention to provide effective interactions to aid the child's development.

The National Autistic Society has a screen tool for adults developed by the Great Manchester consortium which primary care professionals can use. It is available at: www.autism.org.uk/working-with/health/screening-and-diagnosis/screening-measure-for-autism-in-adults.aspx

CONDITIONS ASSOCIATED WITH AN ASC
Sensory problems

Often sensory inputs can appear faulty, leading a person with an ASC to have a considerably confusing experience of the world. Many people with ASC have apparent oversensitive or even painful responses to certain sounds, touch, textures, tastes and smells. This may cause challenging behaviour to everyday noises or even to wearing clothes. In some people they may appear oversensitive to light touch but able to tolerate injuries that would be expected to cause severe pain. Similarly, some people with ASC appear under-sensitive to sensory inputs such as temperature and may apparently feel extreme cold ambient temperatures.

Intellectual disability

Patients with profound intellectual disability have higher prevalence of ASC, presenting considerable challenges to carers along with a higher prevalence of seizures. Intellectual disability occurs in 70% of people with autistic disorder. The other 30% who have a normal range of IQ frequently experience major difficulties in functioning independently, and on intelligence testing the profile may be uneven with advanced visuomotor skills and delayed verbal performance.

Epilepsy

Thirty-eight per cent of children with ASC develop seizures, often starting either in early childhood or adolescence. The high rate of co-occurrence of these disorders may be due to potentially shared underlying mechanisms. Several genetic disorders share epilepsy and autism as prominent phenotypic features, including tuberous sclerosis, Rett syndrome, and fragile X.

Psychiatric disorders

Fifty per cent of those with ASC suffer emotional and behavioural problems. Depression anxiety and psychosis may emerge during adolescence and continue into adulthood.

Fragile X syndrome

This disorder is the most common inherited form of intellectual disability and affects 5% of people with ASC. Fifteen per cent of people with fragile X syndrome will concurrently have an ASC. If a child with ASC also has fragile X, there is a 50% chance that boys born to the same parents will have the syndrome. (*See* Chapter 27.)

Tuberous sclerosis

Tuberous sclerosis is a rare genetic disorder that causes benign tumours to grow in the brain as well as in other vital organs such as the heart, kidney, eyes, lungs and skin. It has a consistently strong association with ASC. One to four per cent of people with ASC also have tuberous sclerosis. (*See* Chapter 29.)

MANAGEMENT

While there is no cure, it remains important to start behavioural interactions and interventions as early as possible. A multidisciplinary team approach is important to coordinate treatments to the specific needs of the child with an ASC and their family and carers.

Behavioural interventions

Therapists and educators can use highly structured and intensive skill-oriented training sessions to help children develop social and language skills, such as applied behavioural analysis, from the age of three. Intensive interaction is a technique using body language to reach people with ASC. It is important to look after the carers and particularly the families and siblings of children and adults with ASC as they manage the challenges and stresses imposed by having someone with ASC.

Medications

Medications can be used for treatment of specific ASD-related symptoms, such as anxiety, depression or obsessive-compulsive disorder, but they are usually unlicensed in the UK. Low-dose SSRIs such as sertraline and fluoxetine are useful to treat anxiety in adolescents with ASC but need regular monitoring. Antipsychotic medications such as risperidone and olanzapine are used to treat severe behavioural problems but require specialist advice. Anticonvulsant drugs are useful in seizure control and prevention.

Other therapies

There have been several false dawns with a number of controversial therapies or interventions available for people with ASC. However, few of these have any evidence base. Parents should use caution before adopting any unproven treatments. Although dietary interventions have been helpful in some children, such as a gluten-free, casein-free diet, carers and healthcare professionals need to ensure an adequate balanced diet is maintained.

OUTCOME

Symptoms can improve with age as the person with ASC changes. However, epilepsy starting in adolescence can compromise this improvement. The best outcomes are in those with higher IQs and those who have acquired spoken language by the age of five.

FURTHER READING

- American Psychiatric Association. *Diagnostic and Statistical Manual of Mental Disorders.* 4th ed., text revision (DSM-IV-TR). APA; 2000.
- Baird G, Simonoff E, Pickles A, *et al.* Prevalence of disorders of the autism spectrum in a population cohort of children in South Thames: the Special Needs and Autism Project (SNAP). *Lancet.* 2006; **368**(9531): 179–81.
- Baron-Cohen S, Scott FJ, Allison C, *et al.* Prevalence of autism-spectrum conditions: UK school-based population study. *Br J Psychiatry.* 2009; **194**: 500–9.
- Danielsson S, Gillberg IC, Billstedt E, *et al.* Epilepsy in young adults with autism: a prospective population-based follow-up study of 120 individuals diagnosed in childhood. *Epilepsia.* 2005; **46**(6): 918–23.
- Dominick KC, Davis NO, Lainhart J, *et al.* Atypical behaviors in children with autism and children with a history of language impairment. *Res Dev Disabil.* 2007; **28**(2): 145–62.
- Filipek PA, Accardo PJ, Baranek GT, *et al.* The screening and diagnosis of autistic spectrum disorders. *J Autism Dev Disord.* 1999; **29**(6): 439–84.
- Lintas C, Persico CM. Autistic phenotypes and genetic testing: state-of-the-art for the clinical geneticist. *J Med Genet.* 2009; **46**: 1–8.
- Millward C, Ferriter M, Calver SJ, *et al.* Gluten- and casein-free diets for autistic spectrum disorder. *Cochrane Database Syst Rev.* 2008; **2**: CD003498.

- Prevalence of autism spectrum disorders – Autism and Developmental Disabilities Monitoring Network (US). *MMWR*. 2009; **58**(SS10): 1–20.
- US Department of Health and Human Services, Public Health Service, National Institutes of Health, National Institute of Child Health and Human Development. *Families and Fragile X Syndrome*; 2003.
- World Health Organization. WHO International Classification of Disease ICD-10 Version 2007.

CHAPTER 27

Fragile X syndrome

Fragile X syndrome is the most commonly known inherited cause of intellectual disability and has a wide variety of presentations. Although caused by a mutation on the X chromosome, it has significant clinical effects in both males and females.

AETIOLOGY
Genetics

Fragile X syndrome is caused by a gene mutation at the fragile X mental retardation 1 (FMR1) gene on the long arm of the X chromosome. Upon culture in a folate-free medium, the affected site has a gap on karyotyping and looks pinched or fragile.

The FMR1 gene produces a protein, FMR1 protein (FMRP), whose function is unknown but thought to be necessary for normal neurological development. Most

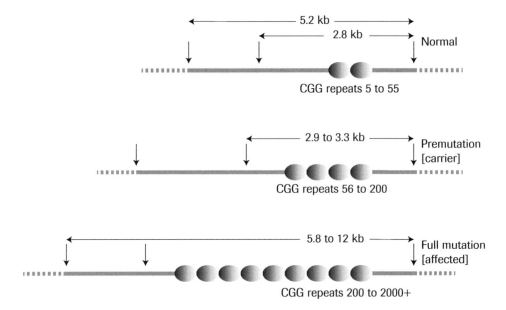

FIGURE 27.1 Diagram of gene and repeat sequence (courtesy of Fragile X Alliance)

people have a normal trinucleotide (cytosine-guanine-guanine [CGG]) repeat sequence of between 6 to 50, with an average of 30 repeats. The mutation is an expansion in the size of this repeating sequence; *see* Figure 27.1 for more details. Expansion only occurs when transmitted through females. The FMR1 gene methylates at more than 200 nucleotide repeats and thus switches off production of FMRP. The features of fragile X syndrome are variable (*see* Table 27.1).

TABLE 27.1 Variable presentation of fragile X syndrome

Number of repeats	Mutation	Effect	Estimates of prevalence in the general population
50 to 200 (females)	Premutation	Usually unaffected carriers	1 in 259 women
50 to 200 (males)	Premutation	Usually unaffected carriers	1 in 755 men
>200 (females)	Full mutation	At least half are affected	1 in 5000 to 8000 females
>200 (males)	Full mutation	Generally affected	1 in 2500 to 4000 males

Pattern of inheritance

Either the man or the woman who carries the affected X chromosome transmits fragile X syndrome premutation or full mutation:

➤ A man with fragile X syndrome premutation will pass it on to all of his daughters without it changing in size, but to none of his sons, as they receive their father's Y chromosome.

➤ A woman with fragile X syndrome premutation will have a 50% chance of passing it on to her sons and daughters, and it is likely to have expanded to a full mutation. The degree of expansion is dependent on the number of repeats.

➤ A woman with a full mutation will pass the full mutation on to 50% of her sons and daughters.

Once an individual is identified with fragile X syndrome, the inheritance will be from the mother, who may carry a premutation or a full mutation. A large proportion of the extended family across generations will be found to carry the premutation, and there may be other affected family members; *see* Figure 27.2. Genetic counselling is important and allows families to make informed decisions about family planning.

PRESENTATION
Individuals with full mutation

Males with the full mutation of the fragile X gene demonstrate developmental, physical, behavioural and emotional characteristics. Females may be affected despite the X linkage, but are usually less affected than males because one of their X chromosomes is unaffected.

Typical features of fragile X syndrome vary in severity and may not always be present. Hence, the absence of typical signs should not deter one from requesting a DNA test to confirm the diagnosis.

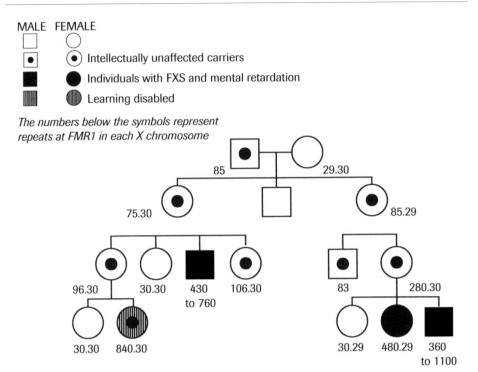

MALE FEMALE

☐ ○

▣ ◉ Intellectually unaffected carriers

■ ● Individuals with FXS and mental retardation

▦ ◍ Learning disabled

The numbers below the symbols represent repeats at FMR1 in each X chromosome

FIGURE 27.2 Diagram of a genogram (courtesy of Fragile X Alliance)

Developmental disability

➤ **Speech disturbances**: speech delay after two years of age, and semantic-pragmatic disorder, are typical, along with other speech disturbances; *see* 'Behavioural and emotional characteristics', (p. 219).

➤ **Intellectual disability**: most males and 30% to 50% of females will have intellectual disability (IQ<70). Intellectual disability varies from mild to severe, with most in the mild to moderate range.

➤ **Other features**: fine and gross motor difficulties, coordination problems, hypotonia. Most females have social anxiety or shyness and learning difficulties.

Physical characteristics

The physical characteristics of large or prominent ears, long face and/or macro-orchidism are seen in up to 80% of males. These features may not be seen before puberty. A high, broad forehead, elongated face, a high, arched palate and man-dibular prognathism may be present. The facial features may be less prominent in women, particularly in those who do not have associated intellectual disability.

Medical conditions

Up to 20% of people with fragile X syndrome have epilepsy, usually tonic-clonic or complex partial seizures.

An elastin disorder associated with fragile X syndrome is thought to explain the following fragile X characteristics – mitral valve prolapse, aortic root dilation, orthopaedic problems (particularly pes planus, hyperextensible joints, pectus exca-vatum, scoliosis, congenital hip dislocation), strabismus and errors of refraction, recurrent ear infections.

Behavioural and emotional characteristics

The so-called 'behavioural phenotype' is often the presenting feature as the physical and developmental issues may be subtle or overlooked. Behavioural and emotional characteristics include:

➤ Attention deficit disorders, with or without hyperactivity. They are common and are demonstrated by distractibility, impulsivity, hyperkinesis and short attention span.

➤ Speech disturbances including variable pitch, perseverative speech (repetition of a word or phrase) and cluttering (rapid speech with repetitions and tangential remarks).

➤ Distinctive hand mannerisms (e.g. hand- and wrist-biting, hand-flapping).

➤ Autistic-like behaviour such as social avoidance and anxiety, stereotypic behaviours, preoccupation with objects, echolalia. Many of the other features of autism such as marked social indifference and severely disturbed interpersonal relationships are, however, rare.

➤ Poor eye contact and gaze aversion, particularly when greeting people. In men, this may be displayed by extending the hand for a handshake while simultaneously turning away the head and trunk.

➤ Sensory defensiveness (e.g. aversion to touch, loud noises, bright lights, strong smells).

➤ Emotional instability (e.g. a tendency towards outbursts of anger and aggression, especially in post-pubertal males).

➤ Hyperarousal or anxiety as prominent features.

Individuals with premutation (fragile X syndrome carriers)

Carriers of fragile X syndrome are generally considered to be unaffected; carrier status is only detected by DNA testing. However, a number of subgroups demon-strate some features of the full mutation, and the term 'short expansion' may be appropriate in these. These subgroups may in fact have a phenotype typical of the fragile X syndrome full mutation, but more subtle. Intellectual disability, executive function defects, anxiety, and mood disorders are often apparent and should be enquired about. A higher incidence of premature ovarian failure has been shown to occur in up to 20% of females carrying the premutation. This has significant implications in terms of offering counselling to older girls and younger women who may wish to start families earlier rather than later. Female premutation may have a higher incidence of chronic affective disorders, schizotypal personality disorders and premature ovarian failure.

Fragile X tremor ataxia syndrome (FXTAS) has recently been described in older males with the premutation. FXTAS is a degenerative neurological disorder demon-strated in approximately 30% of male premutation carriers over the age of 80 years. Males over the age of 50 years presenting with tremor, ataxia, cognitive decline and Parkinson-like deterioration therefore should be asked if there is a family history of fragile X syndrome or developmental delay, and they need to be referred for neuro-logical opinion regardless of family history of fragile X syndrome. Pharmacological management may be helpful. MRIs may confirm the presence of typical lesions in the middle cerebellar peduncles and adjacent white matter.

TESTING

Testing for fragile X syndrome using DNA studies is highly sensitive and specific, and also reliably detects premutation carriers. As the test requires a particular (folate-deficient) medium, when ordering the test specify 'DNA studies for fragile X syndrome'.

Occasionally, fragile X syndrome occurs concomitantly with other syndromes or disabilities (e.g. Down syndrome, cerebral palsy, Pierre Robin syndrome, Prader-Willi syndrome). DNA studies for fragile X syndrome are necessary to confirm the diagnosis of fragile X syndrome.

Cytogenetic testing (karyotyping) is a second test, necessary to detect any other genetic conditions that may be present (e.g. XXY in males).

Who should be tested for fragile X syndrome?

Current international guidelines suggest any individual with significant developmental delay should be tested for fragile X syndrome. The Human Genetics Society of Australasia (HGSA) specify the following indications for DNA testing:

➤ any male or female with intellectual disability (borderline to severe) of unknown cause
➤ individuals with intellectual disability who have had a previous fragile X cytogenetic test that was negative or inconclusive
➤ individuals with a confirmed family history of fragile X syndrome who could have inherited the mutant gene
➤ individuals with learning difficulties of unknown cause, and emotional or behavioural features of fragile X syndrome (including autistic features, anxiety syndromes and attention deficit hyperactivity disorder)
➤ women who experience premature menopause (menopause before the age of 40 years)
➤ adult males (over 50 years of age) who present with unexplained ataxia and/or essential tremor, parkinsonism and dementia.

Refer the family for genetic counselling if an individual tests positive for the fragile X mutation or premutation. If the affected individual is male, genetic testing focuses on his mother and her relatives. Non-affected brothers may carry premutations. It is more common for the premutation to have been inherited from the maternal grandfather than the maternal grandmother.

Cascade testing

Following up family members for testing is known as 'cascade testing', and it needs to be done assiduously; the family GP is ideally suited to be responsible for ensuring this follow-up has occurred.

MANAGEMENT

Specific treatment and intervention strategies are now available and are of great benefit to affected individuals and their families. These include educational, behavioural, pharmacological and medical strategies that integrate multiple professionals as well as the parents and other support persons.

Counselling

Knowledge of genetic issues is important for families and individuals affected by fragile X syndrome. However, an important part of the clinician's role must always be to offer hope and a positive outlook. It needs to be recognised both that families cope well if given sufficient information and support, and that all individuals have an important place in society.

Recommendation

➤ Refer families for genetic counselling.
➤ Institute grief and anger counselling for family members; this should address issues such as loss of expectations.
➤ Ensure that the affected individuals are referred for appropriate assessment, intervention and management.

Early intervention

Being aware of the needs specific to this condition helps affected individuals achieve an optimal outcome. Although most males and some females require lifelong supervision, most individuals achieve good functional life skills.

Support for families

Social supports are important for the families who have a member with fragile X syndrome. The family may need the assistance of a community or social worker to assist not only with personal support but also with accessing financial assistance through applications for pensions and disability allowances. The demands and stresses placed on the families of a person with fragile X syndrome can be immense, especially where the affected person exhibits problem behaviours. Families should be treated with an understanding of the difficulties they may face and be respected for their ability to manage what may be an extremely difficult situation.

Specific issues

Regular review is recommended to detect and manage the wide range of medical issues associated with fragile X syndrome. In addition to genetic counselling and appropriate follow-up, medical practitioners are in the unique position of being able to coordinate pharmacological with behavioural management.

There are no controlled studies on the use of psychotropic medication in the fragile X syndrome population, but these medications are, however, widely used in clinical practice and less rigorous studies provide some evidence to support their use.

There are two main areas requiring behavioural management in people with fragile X syndrome – sensory defensiveness (which can lead to hyperarousal) and attention problems – both of which need to be understood to coordinate behavioural and pharmacological management.

Sensory defensiveness

Sensory defensiveness is the overly sensitive response to touch, smell, sound, sight and taste, which leads to overstimulation or hyperarousal. It requires behavioural management as it may interfere with the ability to take part in learning or social situations. Occupational therapists can develop a sensory diet for the individual (such as appropriate stimulatory or calming activities) to modify responses to sensory overload. The goal is to help the person develop more adaptive responses to the changes and challenges of daily living.

Anxiety and hyperarousal

Anxiety and hyperarousal are major features of fragile X syndrome. Individuals with fragile X syndrome often satisfy the DSM-IV criteria for diagnosis of anxiety disorders, such as panic, generalised anxiety and social anxiety disorders. Treatment of the behavioural components of hyperarousal includes providing a sensory diet, visual cues to transitions or change and the use of appropriate distractors. The majority of cases respond well to SSRIs, selective noradrenaline reuptake inhibitors (SNRIs) and clonidine. *See also* Chapter 13, 'Medication and Challenging Behaviour' (p. 110).

Attention problems

Attention disorders (with or without hyperactivity) always need to be enquired about, as they are very common. They respond to both behavioural and pharmacological management. Behavioural techniques include the use of a sensory diet. Pharmacological options (e.g. methylphenidate or dexamphetamine) produce improvement in most individuals.

Aggression

Aggression, which tends to be more common after the onset of puberty, requires behavioural intervention. Pharmacological interventions including SSRIs, mood stabilisers and risperidone may be useful. *See also* Chapter 12, 'Challenging Behaviour' (p. 93) and Chapter 13, 'Medication and Challenging Behaviour' (p. 103).

Epilepsy and seizure disorders

Epilepsy and seizure disorders are commonly associated with fragile X syndrome. An EEG is mandatory but may not always detect complex partial seizures. Treatment may need to be instituted on clinical impression. Carbamazepine is commonly used in fragile X syndrome, perhaps because of the additional behavioural effects. *See also* Chapter 16, 'Epilepsy' (p. 137).

Mood disorders

Mood disorders occur especially after the onset of puberty. Depression may occur as the individual develops insight, or independently of it. The newer range of SSRIs may be effective. *See also* information on antidepressants in Chapter 15, 'Management of Psychiatric Disorders' (p. 128).

Referrals

To optimise the lives of the affected individuals and their families, it is vital to refer patients to practitioners familiar with fragile X syndrome management issues, so that early implementation of various strategies is possible.

Speech and language therapy, special education, occupational therapy, and clinical and educational psychology may all be needed to allow for the most effective management.

Poor short-term memory, difficulty with auditory processing, abstract concepts, poor attention span and difficulty with initiation all contribute to the academic difficulties affected individuals have. However, affected individuals have a number of strengths that may be capitalised upon to optimise learning and the development of real-life performance skills. These strengths are described in the next section.

Maximising strengths

Individuals with fragile X syndrome generally exhibit many strengths, such as a marvellous sense of humour, socially engaging nature, strong imitation skills, excellent visual skills, visual memory and intense interests. Affected individuals are strong visual learners who do well with pictures and logos, and in particular they learn well with interactive multimedia computer programs. They use their imitation skills and good long-term memory to advantage in drama. They do best with concrete relevant tasks (e.g. shopping and cooking).

In general, individuals with fragile X syndrome thrive in an environment that:

➤ is highly structured and follows routines
➤ has clearly emphasised preparations for changes
➤ includes written and visual schedules to outline the day's activities
➤ has minimal auditory and visual distractions
➤ utilises maximum visual input (such as pictures or drama)
➤ utilises calculators and computers (with interactive multimedia) as teaching tools
➤ involves regular communication between the parent and school.

FURTHER READING

* Braden ML. *Fragile: handle with care*. Revised edition. Colorado Springs: Spectra Publishing Co. Inc.; 2000.
* Metcalf S, Cohen J. Fragile X syndrome – clinical and molecular aspects. 2004. Interactive CD for health professionals and students available from the Fragile X Alliance Inc.: www.fragilex. org.au (accessed 2 February 2011).

CHAPTER 28

Prader-Willi syndrome

Prader-Willi syndrome is a complex genetic condition characterised by neurological impairments causing an altered pattern of growth and development, with hyperphagia (excessive eating). This preoccupation with food and accompanying compulsion to eat can cause extreme obesity and premature death. Lifelong interventions by a multidisciplinary team (including a dietician to prevent excessive weight gain) are crucial. Although there are reports of people living into their eighth decade, there is still significantly increased morbidity and mortality. Most adults live with family or in accommodation with formal support networks.

The condition is mostly sporadic, affecting both males and females, and is not associated with any racial, ethnic or socioeconomic group. Estimates of the birth prevalence vary between 1 in 8500 to 1 in 38 000. It is probable there are many undiagnosed cases of Prader-Willi syndrome.

AETIOLOGY

Prader-Willi syndrome is caused by a lack of expression of paternally contributed genes in a critical region of the long arm of chromosome 15. The Prader-Willi syndrome chromosome region (PWCR) is near the recently isolated candidate gene for Angelman syndrome.

The main genetic mechanisms that have been identified are deletions (70%), maternal uniparental disomy (20% to 30%), translocations, inversions and duplications (5%) and imprinting centre mutations.

PATHOLOGY

Little is known about the neurological pathology leading to congenital hypotonia, growth and metabolic disorders, developmental disability and hyperphagia. There are probably impairments of neurotransmitters and receptors, resulting in multisystem disorders with a variable expression. The hypothalamus is involved, and hyperphagia may be related to an impaired and delayed satiety response due to reduced specific oxytocin neurones (putative satiety cells) in the hypothalamic paraventricular nucleus.

PRESENTATION

Most people with Prader-Willi syndrome come to the attention of doctors because of neonatal hypotonia, developmental delay, intellectual disability, or obesity associated with hyperphagia. The patient may have only one or two of these features.

Until recently the diagnosis was dependent on a scoring system of clinical major and minor criteria and supportive findings. The majority of children with Prader-Willi syndrome are now diagnosed in their first year of life, and the core criteria raising suspicion at birth are the result of the central generalised hypotonia:
➤ floppiness at birth
➤ weak cry or inactivity
➤ poor sucking ability
➤ feeding difficulties
➤ hypogonadism (in boys).

For older children and adults where there is not a reliable neonatal or early history, a high index of suspicion is raised when there are two pervasive characteristics:
➤ hyperphagia
➤ impairments in social cognition, flexibility, abstract ideas and concepts of time and number – even when IQ>70
➤ abnormality in growth – short stature, small hands and feet, hypotonia, narrow forehead.

Hypogonadism is common, and puberty is often delayed.

DIAGNOSIS

A blood test using methylation analysis is used to diagnose Prader-Willi syndrome; the same blood test is also recommended as a screening test. This DNA test distinguishes between the maternal (methylated) and paternal (non-methylated) Prader-Willi syndrome region of chromosome 15.

Further genetic investigations are required to determine the genetic mechanism:
➤ banded cytogenetic analysis – to exclude structural chromosomal anomalies such as translocations
➤ fluorescent *in situ* hybridisation (FISH) – to detect a deletion.

Deletions and maternal disomy are sporadic with no risk of recurrence.

If there is no evidence of a translocation or deletion, maternal disomy can be confirmed by using DNA polymorphism (15 polymerase chain reaction [PCR]) analysis on the patient and their parents.

If all these tests are negative, referral to a geneticist is required to test for an imprinting centre mutation and other rare anomalies.

MANAGEMENT OF ASSOCIATED HEALTH PROBLEMS

In spite of interventions there is considerable morbidity and premature mortality in patients with Prader-Willi syndrome. The health problems are related to hypotonia, altered metabolism, complications of obesity, psychiatric disorders, sleep disorders and other factors. Premature death is commonly associated with cardiorespiratory complications of obesity. Sudden death is not uncommon, and may be related to undiagnosed coronary artery disease or other acute diseases (e.g. peritonitis secondary to a ruptured appendix) that are unrecognised because of a high pain threshold.

Table 28.1 (p. 230) provides an age-related health checklist for people with Prader-Willi syndrome.

Respiratory problems

Hypotonia increases the risk of respiratory disease in young children and adults. Minor upper respiratory infections in young children may cause a croup-like illness with upper airway obstruction. People with Prader-Willi syndrome recover slowly from lower respiratory infections. Recurrent respiratory infections are very common in adults.

Sleep disorders

Intrinsic sleep disorders are increasingly being recognised in people with Prader-Willi syndrome. These include excessive daytime sleeping with an abnormality of the circadian rhythm of rapid eye movement sleep, which is probably due to hypothalamic dysfunction. There are also reports of abnormal responses to hypoxia and hypercapnia; both hypoxia and hypercapnia can be exacerbated by obesity. These factors increase the risk of obstructive sleep apnoea and sleep-related alveolar hypoventilation. A detailed history, with a sleep diary, assists in making the diagnosis, and formal sleep studies (where available) are recommended. There are recent case reports of respiratory deaths in young children.

Short stature

Prader-Willi syndrome is characterised by impaired linear growth. Impaired linear growth, abnormal body composition and hypothalamic dysfunction suggest growth hormone deficiency; however, the research in this area is not conclusive, and not all patients with Prader-Willi syndrome who have short stature have a classical growth hormone deficiency.

Use of growth hormone

Early referral to an endocrinologist is important to discuss the benefits and risks of growth hormone. Regular monitoring of height is essential to detect short stature and a reduction in growth velocity, and if they occur, referral for consideration of growth hormone is recommended.

Growth hormone administered to patients with Prader-Willi syndrome improves height and height velocity in the short term. There is a similar initial improvement in body composition, but the studies looking at quality of life and physical strength are limited. Further international studies are required to determine the role of growth hormone in Prader-Willi syndrome.

Obesity

There is an extreme risk of obesity due to preoccupation with food, low energy expenditure and reduced activity. Obesity increases the risk of diabetes, coronary artery disease, cor pulmonale, sleep apnoea and premature death. Prevention of obesity is of paramount importance for physical, psychological and social well-being and requires sustained lifelong intervention.

It is essential that healthy eating habits be established in the preschool years with supports and interventions maintained throughout life.

Preoccupation with food

All people with Prader-Willi syndrome have a preoccupation with food accompanied by reduced appetite control. Currently, there is no specific drug to counteract this, but fluoxetine and other SSRIs which are useful in obsessive-compulsive disorders show promise. Further research is needed, however, particularly given the association of SSRIs with weight gain.

Low energy expenditure

There is low energy expenditure in people with Prader-Willi syndrome and they require considerably fewer kilojoules than other people. This is partly because patients with Prader-Willi syndrome have a significantly higher proportion of body fat relative to lean body mass than the general population. This decreased fat-free mass is more pronounced in boys than girls, and may reflect early infancy androgen deficiency caused by hypogonadotrophic hypogonadism.

Reduced physical activity

Hypotonia with reduced muscle bulk and strength persists into adult life and contributes to poor posture and reduced stamina for physical activities.

Prevention and management of obesity

Prevention and management of obesity is dependent on a combination of a low kilojoule diet, modification of eating behaviours and participation in regular physical activities. It is essential to establish healthy eating patterns and a low kilojoule diet prior to the onset of the preoccupation with food; parents often need support to do this. They may also need support to convince extended family and community members of the importance of consistency in the approach they have taken. Children and young adults often articulate their difficulties in resisting available food and comment on how they can resist food if they are supervised. The close involvement of a dietician and a psychologist or social worker is useful to maintain nutritional guidelines and strategies throughout a person's life. This is particularly important in residential, vocational or recreational settings, where there is a high turnover of support staff. Generic weight loss strategies that supply specialised diets (such as Weight Watchers) have been useful for some young adults.

RECOMMENDATIONS

➤ Monitor growth and weight – children and adolescents should have their growth regularly measured (and plotted on growth charts to detect early weight gain), and height velocity monitored.
➤ Maintain weight (ideally) at less than the 90th percentile.
➤ Weigh adults regularly and maintain their body mass index (BMI) at less than 25. Monthly to quarterly weighing is usually all that is necessary unless there is rapid weight gain or foraging for food.

All patients need a dietician who can assist in planning and regularly reviewing individualised nutritional guidelines.

Dietary guidelines are essential in all settings (e.g. child care, kindergarten, school, work and home).

DIETARY GUIDELINES

The diet should contain a variety of healthy foods including bread and cereals (including whole grain), vegetables, fruit, minimum-fat milk (or alternatives for adults), and moderate amounts of lean meat or alternatives. The following practices should be promoted.

➤ Avoid foods and drinks high in fat and/or sugar.
➤ Drink water to quench thirst.
➤ Substitute fruit for fruit juice.
➤ Give a list of fat-free foods (such as celery, cucumber, carrot sticks and pickled gherkin) to people involved in the individual's life (e.g. friends, educators).
➤ Establish regular times for meals and snacks.

MODIFICATION OF EXCESSIVE EATING

The total involvement of family and other support persons is essential to ensure the restricted access to food that allows for dietary control. Specific measures need to be taken (such as having an inaccessible pantry, and supervising snacks and meals at school and elsewhere) to restrict opportunities to overeat. It is important to explain the eating disorder and diet programme to extended family, support persons, teachers, employers and others who have contact with the patient. (Provide written individualised information with the general information where appropriate.)

PHYSICAL ACTIVITIES

Exercise and physical activities need to be incorporated into daily life. Physical training programmes can result in increased spontaneous physical activity in people with Prader-Willi syndrome; such training programmes are highly recommended.

BIO-PSYCHOSOCIAL ISSUES

The combination of cognitive difficulties, specific behavioural and personality traits, hyperphagia and interventions that can restrict autonomy cause significant social handicaps for people with Prader-Willi syndrome. Recent reports have shown differences in the cognitive profiles and psychiatric morbidities in the genetic subtypes (deletion and maternal disomy).

Cognitive disabilities

Specific learning and language disorders may occur with a normal intellect, although the majority of people with Prader-Willi syndrome have an IQ in the mild intellectual disability range, often with greater than expected difficulties in adaptive behaviour.

Some specific disabilities described include:
➤ speech difficulties resulting from both hypotonia and cognitive impairments
➤ short-term memory and sequential processing deficits
➤ language processing problems
➤ difficulties in self-reflection and conceptualisation resulting in reduced capacity for self-monitoring.

Recommendation

➤ Refer the person early to a speech pathologist for assessment, advice and (if appropriate) therapy and ongoing surveillance. Some toddlers and preschool children with expressive language delays benefit from Makaton sign language (*see* p. 35).

➤ Refer the person for a detailed cognitive assessment before school entry to identify the learning profile and specific learning disabilities.

Behavioural phenotype

People with Prader-Willi syndrome are at an increased risk of a cluster of behavioural traits possibly related to specific cognitive impairments. The phenotype includes a preoccupation with food and other obsessive traits, mood lability, impulsiveness, temper tantrums, inactivity, repetitive speech patterns, and relative weakness in social skills and adaptive behaviour. Some children's behaviours may lead to a diagnosis of autism spectrum disorder. The behavioural difficulties often increase with age. During school years, special education and psychological assistance are often required for difficulties in adaptive behaviour. Environmental adaptations may be needed to restrict access to food and hence prevent obesity. Adolescence and early adulthood is frequently a period of emotional lability, defiance, difficulties with socialisation and depression.

Early referral to a psychologist for cognitive and clinical assessment, with appropriate ongoing advice, support and interventions is recommended. Long-term follow-up is beneficial for both the patient and their family.

It is important that young people with Prader-Willi syndrome have an opportunity to meet together to express themselves, and discuss their frustrations and difficulties. Referral to a behavioural psychologist for behavioural intervention may be required. Psychiatric and physical illness should be excluded when serious problems arise or when there is a sudden deterioration in behaviour.

Psychiatric disorders

There is an increased risk of psychiatric disease in adults with Prader-Willi syndrome. Recent reports have noted a relationship between family stress and behavioural symptomatology, with a high risk for obsessive compulsive disorders and an increased vulnerability to psychotic disorders.

After excluding or treating any psychiatric disorder, an eclectic approach is required that has a wide range of supports and interventions for behavioural difficulties; it may include pharmacological, behavioural and psychotherapeutic strategies.

TABLE 28.1 Health checklist for people with Prader-Willi syndrome

Life stage	Health issue	Frequency of monitoring	Comments
All age groups	Diet and regular exercise	Each visit*	
	Dental review	Annually	
	Weight	Each visit*	
Infancy	Diagnosis	As early as possible	Include health issues for 'all age groups' (*see above*)
	Genetic counselling		
	Hip ultrasound or X-ray	Each visit*	
	Screening for strabismus	Each visit*	
	Screening for hearing loss		
Toddler and preschool years	Valgus of feet	Annually	Include health issues for 'all age groups' (*see above*)
	Hypogonadism	Annually	
	Vision and hearing	Each visit*	
	Speech	Each visit*	
Childhood	Growth and development	Each visit*	Include health issues for 'all age groups' (*see above*) Refer to endocrinologist for consideration of growth hormone if growth velocity reduced
Primary school	Behavioural difficulties	Annually	Include health issues for 'all age groups' (*see above*)
	Learning difficulties	Annually	Specific investigations and interventions include X-ray and orthopaedic review for scoliosis, treatment of skin infections secondary to skin picking, and the use of SSRIs for skin picking
	Hypogonadism	Annually	
	Scoliosis	Annually	
	Sleep disorders	Annually	A child psychiatrist and behavioural psychologist should be involved in managing behavioural difficulties
	Skin picking	Annually	

Life stage	Health issue	Frequency of monitoring	Comments
Adolescence	Scoliosis Delayed puberty Sleep disorders Skin picking Psychiatric disorders Behavioural problems	Each visit	Include health issues for 'all age groups' (*see above*)
Adults	Skin picking Osteoporosis Diabetes[†] Sleep disorders Ischaemic heart disease[‡] Osteoarthritis Behavioural problems Psychiatric disorders		Include health issues for 'all age groups' (*see above*) Consider hormone replacement therapy for incomplete puberty, osteoporosis or symptoms of menopause and perimenopause Bone mineral density should be measured if there has been a fracture with minimal trauma or there are risk factors

* Each visit (unless specified otherwise) refers to six-monthly reviews with a specialist Prader-Willi syndrome clinic or GP.

† Screening should be performed using fasting plasma glucose. For the general population, screening should be offered to those with a BMI$\geq$30kg/m² if aged 45–54 years, or anyone over 55 years. Given the high prevalence of diabetes in people with Prader-Willi syndrome, screening should be considered for all adult patients with Prader-Willi syndrome. (Butler JV, Whittington JE, Holland AJ, *et al*. Prevalence of, and risk factors for, physical ill-health in people with Prader-Willi syndrome: a population-based study. *Dev Med Child Neurol.* 2002; **44**(4): 248–55.)

‡ While there is scant evidence for a specific association between Prader-Willi syndrome and premature arteriosclerosis, vigilance by clinicians is justified by the association of the syndrome with diabetes and obesity. (Wallace RA. Risk factors for coronary artery disease among individuals with rare syndrome intellectual disability. *J Pol Pract Intellect Disabil.* 2004; **1**(1): 42–51.)

Prader-Willi associations are a valuable source of information and support for parents, professionals and other interested persons. They have a wide range of written materials available for loan and distribution, including specific topics for parents, siblings, teachers, community groups and allied health professionals.

FURTHER READING

- Greenswag LR, Alexander RC, editors. *Management of Prader-Willi Syndrome.* 2nd ed. New York: Springer-Verlag; 1995.
- James TN, Brown RI. *Prader-Willi Syndrome.* London: Chapman and Hall; 1992. (This book, which has a psychosocial and educational orientation, is based on data and direct experience of 50 Canadian families who have a family member with Prader-Willi syndrome.)
- Nixon GM, Brouillette RT. Sleep and breathing in Prader-Willi syndrome. *Pediatr Pulmonol.* 2002; **34**(3): 209–17.
- Paterson WF, Donaldson MD. Growth hormone therapy in the Prader-Willi syndrome. *Arch Dis Child.* 2003; **88**(4): 283–5.
- Waters J. Babies and Children with Prader-Willi Syndrome: a handbook for parents and carers. Prader-Willi Association (UK). Available at: www.pwsa-uk.demon.co.uk/orderform.htm
- Waters J. A handbook for parents and carers of adults with Prader-Willi syndrome. Revised edition. Prader-Willi Association (UK); 1996. Available at: www.pwsa-uk.demon.co.uk/orderform.htm

CHAPTER 29

Tuberous sclerosis

Tuberous sclerosis is characterised clinically by three classical features: intellectual disability, epilepsy and the 'butterfly-shaped' facial rash of angiofibromatas (also known as adenoma sebaceum). It is a multisystem genetic disease in which there are tuber-like growths in the brain and other major organs (including heart and kidneys). However, there is wide variation in the spectrum and severity of its effects, and some have no obvious signs of the condition.

The prevalence is not clear, but it is estimated in children to be between 1 in 6000 to 1 in 17000.

AETIOLOGY

Tuberous sclerosis is inherited in an autosomal dominant fashion, although sporadic new mutations are responsible for up to two-thirds of cases. Recent advances in molecular genetics have shed additional light on inheritance and pathophysiology. Virtually all cases arise from mutations in either the TSC1 or the TSC2 genes, although it is now appreciated that other genetic – and also environmental – factors influence clinical severity.

DIAGNOSIS

Standardised diagnostic criteria have been developed (see Table 29.1). A neurologist, paediatrician or clinical geneticist usually assesses the patient for the diagnosis with the aid of brain, cardiac and renal imaging, as well as other specialised ophthalmological, dental and skeletal assessments. Examining the child and both parents with a Wood's light (which shows the hypomelanotic patches) is often diagnostically rewarding.

CHARACTERISTICS
Skin lesions

The skin lesions are of a number of types.
➤ The angiofibromas are rarely obvious before the age of two years, and first appear as small erythematous lesions. They often proliferate during puberty and can be confused with acne.
➤ Hypomelanotic patches (depigmented patches; also known as 'ash leaf') are a common sign, occurring in 60% of those affected. These white patches are the

TABLE 29.1 Diagnosis of tuberous sclerosis

Likelihood of having tuberous sclerosis
Definite: two major features, or one major feature plus two minor features
Probable: one major feature plus one minor feature
Possible: one major feature, or two or more minor features

Major features	Minor features
Facial angiofibromas or forehead plaque	Multiple randomly distributed pits in dental
Non-traumatic ungual or periungual	enamel
fibromas	Hamartomatous rectal polyps
Hypomelanotic macules (three or more)	Bone cysts
Shagreen patch (connective tissue nevus)	Cerebral white matter radial migration
Multiple retinal nodular hamartomas	lines†§
Cortical tuber*	Gingival fibromas
Subependymal nodule	Non-renal hamartoma
Subependymal giant cell astrocytoma	Retinal achromic patch
Cardiac rhabdomyoma, single or multiple	'Confetti' skin lesions
Lymphangiomyomatosis†	Multiple renal cysts
Renal angiomyolipoma†	

* Cerebral cortical dysplasia and cerebral white matter migration tracts occurring together are counted as one rather than two features of tuberous sclerosis.

† When both lymphangiomyomatosis and renal angiomyolipomas are present, other features of tuberous sclerosis must be present before tuberous sclerosis is diagnosed.

§ White matter migration lines and focal cortical dysplasia are often seen in patients with tuberous sclerosis; however, because these lesions can be seen independently and are relatively non-specific, they are considered minor diagnostic criteria for tuberous sclerosis.

     first cutaneous abnormality and can usually be detected in infancy and early childhood. Examination under a Wood's light is often required to identify these, especially in fair-skinned individuals and infants.

➤ Shagreen patches (French: chagrin – grained skin) are thickened and raised yellowish areas of skin on the lower back, which occur in approximately half of cases.

➤ Subungual or periungual fibromas occur under and around the fingernails and become more prevalent with age. These lesions cause grooves in the nail and occasionally these are the only signs of tuberous sclerosis.

Seizures

Seizures occur in up to 80% of cases and range in severity from subtle to very severe. Infantile spasms (jackknife or salaam seizures), complex partial seizures and myoclonic seizures are the most common types encountered. The first evidence of tuberous sclerosis may be infantile spasms. Seizures can be difficult to control but may become less of a problem with age.

Intellectual disability

About half of those affected with tuberous sclerosis have associated intellectual disability; the exact figure is, however, debated. There is a definite association between the severity of the intellectual disability and the severity of the epilepsy.

Other health and behavioural issues

There are other issues to note.

➤ Cortical tubers are usually related to the severity of the epilepsy and intellectual disability. Rarely, a cortical tuber may undergo malignant degeneration.

➤ Subependymal hamartomas are markers for the disease, but they do not usually have complications.

➤ The renal cystic disease can be indistinguishable from autosomal dominant polycystic kidney disease and usually presents in infancy. Renal angiomyolipomas tend to present after puberty.

➤ Rhabdomyomata of the heart may cause problems in the perinatal period. Tumours may also occur in the eye, bone, lung and liver.

➤ Sleeping problems are common in children.

➤ Behavioural difficulties are frequent and include hyperactivity (59% of cases), aggressive behaviour (13%) and autism (50%).

➤ Dental abnormalities such as multiple enamel pits are often found, and sometimes assist the diagnostic evaluation.

MANAGEMENT

The management of tuberous sclerosis involves:

➤ genetic counselling for the family (the causative TCS1and TCS2 gene mutations can be found in up to 80% of cases and this introduces the option of future prenatal diagnosis for families)

➤ epilepsy management, particularly as developmental progress may be severely restricted by poorly controlled seizures

➤ treatment of cutaneous lesions with laser therapy, dermabrasion and cautery

➤ specific behavioural management (as required)

➤ regular dental care

➤ five-yearly renal ultrasound scans.

Treatment may also be required for cardiac outflow obstruction or arrhythmias, which may occur in association with rhabdomyomata (particularly in infancy). Occasionally, focal seizures arising from central nervous system hamartomas can be ameliorated by neurosurgical intervention that is guided by specialised neurological studies.

FURTHER READING

• Kandt RS. Tuberous sclerosis: the next step. *J Child Neurol.* 1993; **8**(2): 107–10; discussion 110–11.

• O'Callaghan FJ. Tuberous sclerosis. *BMJ.* 1999; **318**(7190): 1019–20.

• Roach ES, Gomez MR, Northrup H. Tuberous sclerosis complex consensus conference: revised clinical diagnostic criteria. *J Child Neurol.* 1998; **13**(12): 624–8.

• Webb DW, Clarke A, Fryer A, *et al.* The cutaneous features of tuberous sclerosis: a population study. *Br J Dermatol.* 1996; **135**(1): 1–5.

• Webb DW, Osborne JP. Tuberous sclerosis. *Arch Dis Child.* 1995; **72**(6): 471–4.

CHAPTER 30

Rett syndrome

Rett syndrome is a neurodevelopmental disorder seen almost exclusively in females. It was originally described by Andreas Rett in 1966. Severe intellectual and physical handicap are predominant features; however, IQ assessment by traditional methods is difficult.

In Australia, Rett syndrome was found in 1 in 14 000 girls aged between five and 18 years and it has been estimated that, on average, 12 girls will be born each year who will be diagnosed with this disorder by the age of 12 years. Little is known about life expectancy.

AETIOLOGY

Rett syndrome is a genetic disorder and is now known to be caused, in the majority of cases, by mutations in the MECP2 gene. About 99% of cases arising from MECP2 gene mutations are single occurrences in a family as a result of a *de novo* mutation in the child with Rett syndrome. Very rarely, the mother carries the mutation but has been protected from its effects by skewed X inactivation. In such cases, or if the mother has germline mosaicism, there is a risk of another child being born who will develop the disorder.

CLINICAL AND MOLECULAR DIAGNOSIS

The clinical diagnosis of Rett syndrome is challenging because the clinical features necessary for diagnosis only become apparent with time. Although there are well-established criteria, cases are often misclassified early as Angelman syndrome, Prader-Willi syndrome, autism, congenital hypotonia, cerebral palsy, or other (rarer) neurodegenerative disorders. It is likely that there are adults with Rett syndrome who remain undiagnosed or misdiagnosed; this makes it difficult to estimate life expectancy.

There are both necessary and supportive criteria (see below), and also exclusionary criteria (to reduce the likelihood of misclassification). Rett syndrome is diagnosed as 'classical' when all the necessary criteria are present, and 'atypical' when the typical clinical characteristics are seen in the absence of all the necessary criteria. These atypical cases can be further subdivided into 'mild atypical' (have not shown head growth deceleration and are more likely to remain ambulant) and 'early onset atypical' (without normal early development, and usually having a more severe phenotype). In 2002, modifications were suggested to the original criteria to take into account the fact that normal development may be delayed from birth and consequently head circumference growth deceleration may not occur.

Detection of a pathogenic MECP2 mutation is very helpful clinically as it provides independent confirmation of a challenging clinical diagnosis. Failure to find a mutation, however, is not equivalent to excluding the diagnosis, as about 20% of cases have no apparent defect within the gene. There are eight common mutations which account for about two-thirds of cases with MECP2 mutations; some of these mutations are associated with a milder and some a more severe clinical picture.

CHARACTERISTICS
Necessary criteria
The criteria necessary for a diagnosis of Rett syndrome are:
➤ apparently normal prenatal and perinatal period
➤ apparently normal psychomotor development through the first six months of life; however, psychomotor development may be delayed from birth
➤ normal head circumference at birth
➤ deceleration of head growth (in the majority of cases) between five months and four years of age
➤ loss of acquired purposeful hand skills between six and 30 months of age, temporally associated with communication dysfunction and social withdrawal
➤ development of severely impaired expressive and receptive language, and presence of apparent severe psychomotor retardation
➤ stereotypic hand movements (such as wringing, squeezing, clapping, tapping); mouthing, washing and rubbing automatisms appear after purposeful hand skills are lost
➤ appearance of gait apraxia, truncal apraxia and ataxia between ages one and four years
➤ a tentative diagnosis until ages two to five years.

Supportive criteria
Supportive criteria are frequently found characteristics that are supportive of, but not mandatory for, the diagnosis. These include:
➤ breathing abnormalities involving both hyperventilation and periods of apnoea
➤ EEG abnormalities
➤ seizures
➤ scoliosis
➤ vasomotor instability with very cold feet.

Although the slowing of head growth is the only growth parameter listed as one of the necessary criteria, Rett syndrome is now considered to affect many parameters of growth, and hands and feet are typically small. Girls with Rett syndrome are often hypotonic in their early years and later develop spasticity with muscle wasting and characteristic dystonia.

Additional features
Other features that, if present, make the diagnosis more likely include abdominal bloating, teeth grinding, abnormal pain sensation, sleep disturbance, night laughing and eye pointing (communicating with the eyes).

Radiography of the hands and feet can assist with the diagnosis in females over four years of age; this is particularly useful in older girls and adult women as either a short fourth metatarsal or a short ulna is present in over half of this group. Osteopenia and fractures are common.

MANAGEMENT

The management of Rett syndrome involves:

➤ establishing a definitive diagnosis (although distressing, having a diagnosis confirmed is generally valued by parents and family). Not only does the diagnosis provide insight into the cause of the child's clinical features, it also facilitates access to support services

➤ antiepileptic medication (if seizures are present – video EEG monitoring can help with the diagnosis of epilepsy)

➤ nutritional management – sometimes requiring a gastrostomy

➤ physiotherapy – as it has a major role in maintaining ambulation and helping to prevent osteopenia

➤ occupational therapy – to help maintain function and prevent deformities.

Management may also involve:

➤ referral to an orthopaedic specialist. This is often required and is particularly relevant for the monitoring and management of scoliosis; scoliosis often benefits from surgical intervention

➤ active management of constipation (the majority of girls and women with Rett syndrome require this)

➤ music therapy and hydrotherapy (girls with Rett syndrome generally respond well)

➤ communication aids – both simple and more sophisticated.

FURTHER READING

- Amir RE, Zoghbi HY. Rett syndrome: methyl-CpG-binding protein 2 mutations and pheno-type-genotype correlations. *Am J Med Genet.* 2000; **97**(2): 147–52.
- Colvin L, Fyfe S, Leonard S, *et al.* Describing the phenotype in Rett syndrome using a population database. *Arch Dis Child.* 2003; **88**(1): 38–43.
- Hagberg B. Clinical criteria, stages and natural history. In: Hagberg B, editor. *Rett Syndrome: clinical and biological aspects.* London: Mac Keith Press; 1993.
- Hagberg B, Hanefeld F, Percy A, *et al.* An update on clinically applicable diagnostic criteria in Rett syndrome. Comments to Rett Syndrome Clinical Criteria Consensus Panel Leonard H, Bower C, English D. The prevalence and incidence of Rett syndrome in Australia. *Eur Child Adolesc Psychiatry.* 1997; **6**(Suppl. 1): S8–10.
- Satellite to European paediatric neurology society meeting, Baden Baden, Germany, 11 September 2001. *Eur J Paediatr Neurol.* 2002; **6**(5): 293–7.

CHAPTER 31

Williams syndrome

Williams and Barratt-Boyes first described Williams syndrome in New Zealand in 1961.

The epidemiology of Williams syndrome is not well studied, but in Western Australia it occurs in less than 1 in 20 000 births.

AETIOLOGY

It has recently been established that the great majority of Williams syndrome cases occur as a result of a microdeletion on the long arm of chromosome 7, almost always involving the elastin gene (ELN).

A defect in elastin may account for the abnormalities found in connective tissue in the aorta and in the larynx. However, the etiological basis for the cognitive and behavioural problems remains unknown.

DIAGNOSIS

Typically, affected infants have a characteristic facial appearance as well as supravalvular aortic stenosis. Intellectual disability (which can vary in severity) may be masked by an unusually friendly outgoing personality. Presentation in infancy can include failure to thrive, vomiting, and constipation alternating with diarrhoea (often arising from hypercalcaemia). At the time of the initial diagnosis, a series of specialised evaluations is recommended, including complex physical and neurological examinations; plotting of growth parameters on Williams syndrome growth charts; calcium estimation; thyroid function tests; cardiology, urinary system and ophthalmic evaluations; and genetics consultation.

Fluorescent *in situ* hybridisation (FISH) identifies a submicroscopic deletion at 7q11.23 in 95% of cases.

CHARACTERISTICS
Facial features

Commonly seen facial features include:
➤ periorbital fullness
➤ stellate irides
➤ malar hypoplasia
➤ a broad nasal tip with anteverted nares and a full lower lip (often with an open mouth appearance)

➤ sagging cheeks in infancy and childhood – these become thin in adolescence or early adulthood
➤ strabismus.

Characteristic dental anomalies may also occur.

Growth

Williams syndrome may be associated with intrauterine growth retardation. Both children and adults may be short in stature, and microcephaly is often present. Menarche may be early.

Medical issues

There are many associated medical conditions:
➤ cardiac abnormalities in about 75% of cases – the most common reported are supravalvular aortic stenosis and peripheral pulmonary artery stenosis
➤ hypertension – frequently found in adults
➤ myocardial ischaemia associated with stenosis of the left coronary artery
➤ strokes and chronic hemiparesis – associated with stenosis of the cerebral arteries
➤ renal abnormalities in approximately 20% of cases – including bladder diverticulae, renal hypoplasia and duplicated kidneys
➤ urinary tract infections, chronic constipation and diverticulosis
➤ hoarse voice (common)
➤ inguinal hernia – in many children
➤ orthopaedic problems – such as joint contractures and scoliosis
➤ infantile hypercalcaemia – may present as constipation.

Cognitive, behavioural and neurological problems

Infant behaviour is often described as difficult with irritability and poor feeding. Older children tend to be friendly and talkative, and may be socially uninhibited; their intellectual ability may be overestimated because of their apparently good verbal skills.

Cognitive deficits vary from mild to moderate intellectual disability, with perceptual and motor function more reduced than verbal and memory performance. Emotional and behavioural disturbances (including generalised anxiety and attention deficit problems) are common; they may improve in adolescence and adulthood. Hyperacusis has also been reported. Hypotonia is frequent in the younger years but progresses later to hypertonia.

MANAGEMENT

The management of Williams syndrome involves:
➤ screening for congenital heart disease and, if identified, subsequent management
➤ urinary system evaluation (including ultrasound screening of the renal system)
➤ ophthalmological review
➤ regular dental care
➤ physiotherapy (in children with musculoskeletal and neurological problems)

➤ regular blood pressure checks in adults, with antihypertensive treatment instituted when necessary.

Feeding, gastrointestinal and urinary problems may also need to be managed, and behavioural difficulties may require psychological intervention.

FURTHER READING

- Ashkenas J. Williams syndrome starts making sense. *Am J Hum Genet*. 1996; **59**(4): 756–61.
- Burn J. Williams syndrome. *J Med Genet*. 1986; **23**(5): 389–95.
- Doctor's resources for Williams syndrome. Williams Syndrome Association. Available at: www. williams-syndrome.org/fordoctors/index.html
- Gosch A, Pankau R. Personality characteristics and behaviour problems in individuals of different ages with Williams syndrome. *Dev Med Child Neurol*. 1997; **39**(8): 527–33.
- Lopez-Rangel E, Maurice M, McGillivray B, *et al*. Williams syndrome in adults. *Am J Med Genet*. 1992; **44**(6): 720–9.

CHAPTER 32

Angelman syndrome

Angelman syndrome is a severe neurodevelopmental disorder associated with intellectual disability. Other features include severe speech impairment, gait ataxia and tremulousness of the limbs, and a distinctive behaviour with an inappropriate happy affect that includes frequent laughing, smiling and excitability. Microcephaly and seizures are common.

The epidemiology of Angelman syndrome has not been widely researched; however, the incidence has been estimated at less than 1 in 10 000 births.

AETIOLOGY

This disorder is now known to be caused by a variety of genetic mechanisms involving chromosome 15. These include deletion of the maternally derived Angelman syndrome locus (75%), paternal uniparental disomy (2%), an imprinting mutation (1%) and UBE3A mutation (11%). Paradoxically, in the small proportion of cases where genetic studies are normal, familial recurrence is high.

DIAGNOSIS

Diagnostic criteria are based on the clinical characteristics summarised below. Clinical diagnosis is difficult in the first two to three years of life. Conditions with a similar presentation include Rett syndrome, Lennox-Gastaut syndrome, autism and non-specific cerebral palsy.

In about 90% of cases, clinical diagnosis can be confirmed by laboratory testing. The cornerstone of diagnosis remains clinical evaluation by a clinician experienced with the nuances of this challenging diagnosis – particularly as 10% of cases cannot be confirmed by laboratory testing. Clinicians who have the greatest familiarity with diagnosing Angelman syndrome are clinical geneticists and developmental paediatricians.

CLINICAL CHARACTERISTICS

The developmental history and findings of investigations include:
- normal antenatal and birth history
- normal head circumference at birth
- an absence of major birth defects
- developmental delay evident by six to 12 months of age with ongoing delay in development (but no regression)

➤ normal metabolic, haematological and chemical laboratory profiles
➤ no structural brain abnormalities.

Table 32.1 shows the characteristics of Angelman syndrome and their chance of being present in individuals.

TABLE 32.1 Clinical characteristics of Angelman syndrome and their incidence

Present in 100% of cases	Present in at least 80% of cases	Present in 20% to 80% of cases
Severe developmental delay Speech impairment with minimal or no use of words Receptive language better than expressive language Movement or balance disorder A distinctive behavioural phenotype that includes: frequent laughter excitability hand-flapping hyperactivity	Absolute or relative microcephaly by the age of two years Seizures with onset usually before the age of three years Characteristic EEG changes	Flat occiput Occipital grooves Deep-set eyes Prominent jaw Wide mouth and widely spaced teeth Tongue thrusting Hypopigmented skin Fair to blond hair Hyperactive lower limb deep tendon reflexes (often difficult to assess) Increased sensitivity to heat Sleep disturbances (which improve with age) Fascination with water

Children with Angelman syndrome can acquire some simple skills associated with daily living but not to the level of being able to live independently. By adulthood, about 80% are toilet-trained by day.

MANAGEMENT

The management of Angelman syndrome involves:
➤ diagnosis, particularly as it provides an explanation for the child's disability; it also gives parents access to the benefits of a support association. Referral to a genetic clinic can be helpful in the diagnostic process
➤ seizure management
➤ specific management of hyperactive behaviour
➤ respite for the family.

Children may also benefit from physiotherapy, and occupational and speech therapy.

FURTHER READING

• Alessandri LM, Leonard H, Blum LM, *et al*. *Disability Counts: a profile of disability in Western Australia*. Perth: Disability Services Commission; 1996.
• Clayton-Smith J, Pembrey ME. Angelman syndrome. *J Med Genet*. 1992; **29**(6): 412–15.
• Petersen MB, Brondum-Nielsen K, Hansen LK, *et al*. Clinical, cytogenetic, and molecular diagnosis of Angelman syndrome: estimated prevalence rate in a Danish county. *Am J Med Genet*. 1995; **60**(3): 261–2.

- Stalker HJ, Williams CA. Genetic counseling in Angelman syndrome: the challenges of multiple causes. *Am J Med Genet.* 1998; **77**(1): 54–9.
- Williams CA, Angelman H, Clayton-Smith J, *et al.* Angelman syndrome: consensus for diagnostic criteria. Angelman Syndrome Foundation. *Am J Med Genet.* 1995; **56**(2): 237–8.

CHAPTER 33

Noonan syndrome

First discovered as a distinct entity in 1963, Noonan syndrome displays considerable variation in expression, and the phenotype changes with age. The cardinal features are short stature, congenital heart disease (predominantly valvular pulmonary stenosis), mild intellectual disability and a characteristic facial appearance with a broad or webbed neck.

The epidemiology of Noonan syndrome remains poorly defined. It has been estimated that Noonan syndrome with intellectual disability accounts for less than 1 in 10 000 births; however, as Noonan syndrome is not always associated with intellectual disability, the true incidence of the syndrome may be much higher.

AETIOLOGY

The pattern of transmission in families suggests autosomal dominant inheritance, although a significant proportion of cases are sporadic. PTPN11 gene mutations are identifiable in approximately 50% of cases.

DIAGNOSIS

Diagnosis, which is based on clinical findings, is usually made by a clinical geneticist or an experienced paediatrician. The differential diagnosis of Noonan syndrome includes Williams syndrome, foetal alcohol syndrome and Aarskog syndrome. There is some overlap between the phenotypes of Noonan and neurofibromatosis, as café au lait patches and pigmented naevi commonly occur in Noonan syndrome. Detection of a pathogenic mutation in the PTPN11 gene provides useful evidence to confirm the diagnosis, particularly in atypical cases.

CHARACTERISTICS

People with Noonan syndrome have characteristic facial features. These include:
➤ hypertelorism (widely spaced eyes)
➤ ptosis
➤ downslanting palpebral fissures
➤ a low posterior hairline
➤ excess nuchal skin – in the newborn
➤ neck webbing – more obvious in older children
➤ triangular contour of the face – as the child gets older.

Other features commonly seen include:
➤ strabismus and refractive errors
➤ low-set and posteriorly rotated ears
➤ a high arched palate
➤ flattened nasal bridge
➤ micrognathia
➤ wispy hair in infancy, which becomes more curly or woolly in the older child.

Growth

Short stature occurs in 80% of individuals with Noonan syndrome. It arises from a prepubertal growth pattern that tends to parallel the 3rd percentile with relatively normal growth velocity. In both sexes puberty may be either normal or delayed. Over half the males with Noonan syndrome have at least one undescended testis, and there may be inadequate secondary sexual development associated with deficient spermatogenesis. The majority of females are fertile.

Medical issues

There are many medical conditions that may be associated with Noonan syndrome:
➤ congenital heart defects – in about two-thirds. Individuals with Noonan syndrome display a typical ECG pattern:
 — pulmonary valvular stenosis representing about half of the cardiac defects
 — atrial septal defect
 — asymmetrical septal hypertrophy
 — ventricular septal defect and persistent ductus arteriosus
➤ chest deformity (such as pectus carinatum, pectus excavatum) – in 90%
➤ cubitus valgus and hand anomalies – common
➤ scoliosis and talipes equinovarus
➤ abnormal bleeding and bruising – approximately one-third of individuals with Noonan syndrome have one or more coagulation defects
➤ unexplained hepatosplenomegaly – in about 25%
➤ abnormalities of the lymphatic channels – sometimes leading to general or peripheral lymphoedema
➤ hypotonia – common.

Seizures, and vision and hearing impairments, have also been reported in children.

Cognitive and behavioural problems

About one-third of individuals with Noonan syndrome have mild intellectual disability with the average IQ being approximately 10 points below that of unaffected family members. The disability appears to be associated with specific visual-constructional problems. Language delay may be secondary to perceptual motor disabilities, mild hearing loss or articulation problems. A behavioural phenotype questionnaire found children with Noonan syndrome to be clumsy, stubborn and irritable; some also experienced psychiatric problems and communication difficulties.

MANAGEMENT

The management of Noonan syndrome involves:

➤ referral to a clinical geneticist to confirm the diagnosis. They can also provide information about both the natural course of Noonan syndrome, and counselling about the inheritance and the risk of recurrence
➤ specialist care and long-term monitoring of any congenital heart disease
➤ screening for clotting abnormalities
➤ assessment and monitoring of hearing and vision, including an audiological and ophthalmological examination
➤ referral and management for cryptoorchidism (if present in males)
➤ treatment for epilepsy (if epilepsy is present)
➤ assessment, and possibly intervention, for specific learning deficits.

FURTHER READING

- Allanson JE. Noonan syndrome. *J Med Genet.* 1987; **24**(1): 9–13.
- Musante L, Kehl HG, Majewski F, *et al.* Spectrum of mutations in PTPN11 and genotype-phenotype correlation in 96 patients with Noonan syndrome and five patients with cardio-facio-cutaneous syndrome. *Eur J Hum Genet.* 2003; **11**(2): 201–6.
- Sharland M, Burch M, McKenna WM, *et al.* A clinical study of Noonan syndrome. *Arch Dis Child.* 1992; **67**(2): 178–83.
- Wood A, Massarano A, Super M, *et al.* Behavioural aspects and psychiatric findings in Noonan's syndrome. *Arch Dis Child.* 1995; **72**(2): 153–5.

CHAPTER 34

Neurofibromatosis type 1

Neurofibromatosis type 1 (NF1) is a distinctive neurocutaneous syndrome that was first described in the late 19th century. Common clinical features include multiple café au lait spots, axillary and inguinal freckling, multiple palpable dermal fibromas, and small tumours on the iris (Lisch nodules). Intellectual disability, which ranges from subtle to severe, occurs commonly. Other manifestations include optic and central nervous system gliomas, plexiform neurofibromas, peripheral nerve sheath tumours, bony lesions and vasculopathy.

Neurofibromatosis type 2 is a much rarer genetic disorder involving suscepti-bility to neuronal tissue overgrowth, typically characterised by bilateral vestibular schwannomas (acoustic neuromas). Because of the rarity of neurofibromatosis type 2, it is not included in this book.

AETIOLOGY

NF1 arises from loss-of-function mutations within the NF1 gene (which encodes neurofibromin, an important regulator of cell growth).

DIAGNOSIS

The diagnosis of NF1 is based on clinical findings that are usually unequivocal in all but a very small proportion of young infants.

Molecular genetic testing is rarely necessary for diagnostic purposes. Once a clinical diagnosis has been established, identification of the causative NF1 gene mutation permits predictive and prenatal testing, when required.

The National Institutes of Health (NIH) diagnostic criteria for NF1 are met in an individual who has two or more of the following features:

➤ six or more café au lait macules that are over 5 mm in greatest diameter in prepubertal individuals, or over 15 mm in greatest diameter in postpubertal individuals
➤ two or more neurofibromas (of any type) or one plexiform neurofibroma
➤ freckling in the axillary or inguinal regions
➤ optic glioma
➤ two or more Lisch nodules (iris hamartomas)
➤ a distinctive osseous lesion such as sphenoid dysplasia or thinning of long bone cortex with or without pseudarthrosis
➤ a first-degree relative with NF1 as defined by the above criteria.

The NIH diagnostic criteria are both highly specific and sensitive in adults with NF1. Only about half of the patients with NF1 and no known family history of neurofibromatosis meet the NIH criteria for diagnosis by one year of age, but almost all do by eight years of age, because many features of NF1 increase in frequency with age.

Segmental or regional neurofibromatosis is sometimes diagnosed in patients who have features of NF1 restricted to only one part of the body.

CHARACTERISTICS

The clinical manifestations of NF1 are extremely variable.

➤ Multiple café au lait spots occur in virtually all cases and associated axillary/inguinal freckling is present in up to 90% of cases.
➤ Neurofibromas may affect virtually any organ in the body. Numerous benign cutaneous neurofibromas are normally present in affected adults. Plexiform neurofibromas, which are less common, may cause disfigurement and compromise function. Ocular manifestations include optic gliomas (which may lead to blindness) and Lisch nodules. Skeletal manifestations include scoliosis, vertebral dysplasia, pseudarthrosis and overgrowth.
➤ Intellectual disability occurs in up to 50% of cases. Children with neurofibromatosis are at an increased risk of attention deficit disorders.
➤ Cardiac complications include pulmonary valvular stenosis and hypertension. Hypertension, which increases in frequency with age, has a range of aetiologies including renal artery stenosis and coarctation of the aorta.
➤ Although most pregnancies in women with NF1 are normal, serious complications have been reported. Women with NF1 may experience an increase in the number and size of neurofibromas during pregnancy; other pregnancy-related complications include hypertension and problems with delivery (which require specialist attention).
➤ Vasculopathy, intracranial tumours, and malignant peripheral nerve sheath tumours are other medical concerns, and increase in frequency with age.
➤ Although there is an increased occurrence of malignancies, they occur in only a minority of cases.

The majority of symptoms arise from local pressure effects of non-malignant over-growths, particularly within the central and peripheral nervous systems.

MANAGEMENT

Because of the many potential complications arising from NF1, specialist medical input is required for management of individuals with the condition. The clinician should seek to obtain:

➤ personal medical history with particular attention to the range of clinical features associated with NF1
➤ family history with particular attention to subtle features of NF1 (clinical geneticists have much to offer)
➤ physical examination with particular focus on the cutaneous, skeletal and neurological systems
➤ ophthalmological evaluation (including slit lamp examination of the irises)
➤ detailed developmental assessment (if a child)

➤ other studies (if indicated on the basis of clinically apparent signs or symptoms).

More extensive investigations are sometimes required, depending on clinical findings, and multidisciplinary input is often required.

The follow-up of patients includes the following:

➤ annual physical examination by a physician who is familiar with the patient and with the disease

➤ annual ophthalmological examination in childhood, and less frequently in adults

➤ regular blood pressure monitoring

➤ other studies as indicated on the basis of clinically apparent signs or symptoms.

The interpretation of neuroimages from patients with NF1 can be highly challenging. Patients can benefit from the professional input of specialist clinicians who are familiar with the full range of clinical complications that may arise in NF1 – especially when surgical intervention is being considered. The clinical decision-making associated with optic gliomas in patients with NF1 is an example of the type of challenge that may be encountered. Most patients with optic nerve tumours detected by MRI remain symptom-free. Furthermore, symptomatic optic nerve lesions in patients with NF1 are usually stable for many years, or only progress very slowly; some lesions may even spontaneously regress in the absence of treatment.

FURTHER READING

- DeBella K, Szudek J, Friedman JM. Use of the national institutes of health criteria for diagnosis of neurofibromatosis 1 in children. *Pediatrics*. 2000; **105**(3/1): 608–14.
- Friedman JM, Riccardi VM. Clinical epidemiological features. In: Friedman JM, Gutmann DH, MacCollin M, Riccardi VM, editors. *Neurofibromatosis: phenotype, natural history, and pathogenesis*. Baltimore: Johns Hopkins University Press; 1999, pp. 29–86.
- Gutmann DH, Aylsworth A, Carey JC, *et al.* The diagnostic evaluation and multidisciplinary management of neurofibromatosis 1 and neurofibromatosis 2. *JAMA*. 1997; **278**(1): 51–7.
- Huson SM. Neurofibromatosis 1: a clinical and genetic overview. In: Huson SM, Hughes RAC, editors. *The Neurofibromatoses: a pathogenetic and clinical overview*. London: Chapman and Hall, pp. 204–32.
- North K. Cognitive function and academic performance. In: Friedman JM, Gutmann DH, MacCollin M, Riccardi VM, editors. *Neurofibromatosis: phenotype, natural history, and pathogenesis*. Baltimore: Johns Hopkins University Press; 1999, pp. 162–89.

CHAPTER 35

Foetal alcohol syndrome

Foetal alcohol syndrome (FAS) is recognised as the leading, preventable, non-genetic cause of intellectual impairment. The teratogenic effects of alcohol produce outcomes that range in severity from full FAS through to milder or less complete forms. 'Foetal alcohol spectrum disorders' is an umbrella term now being used frequently to cover all the foetal effects of alcohol:

➤ foetal alcohol spectrum disorder (a defined group of physical features) with confirmed maternal alcohol exposure
➤ foetal alcohol spectrum disorder without confirmed maternal alcohol exposure
➤ partial foetal alcohol spectrum (not all the physical features of the syndrome) disorder with confirmed maternal alcohol exposure
➤ alcohol-related birth defects of heart, bone, kidney
➤ alcohol-related neurodevelopmental disorder without characteristic physical features.

The birth prevalence of FAS varies between countries, and between ethnic groups within countries. In the UK approx 1% newborn are affected by excess maternal alcohol intake, 0.1% have the full foetal alcohol syndrome and 0.3%–0.4% have foetal alcohol spectrum disorder.

AETIOLOGY

While maternal alcohol consumption during pregnancy can result in foetal alcohol spectrum disorders, not all children exposed to alcohol *in utero* are affected, or are affected to the same extent.

The expression of full FAS results from either a chronic, heavy pattern of maternal alcohol consumption that occurs on a daily basis, or frequent heavy intermittent alcohol use of at least five drinks per occasion at least once a week ('binge drinking'). Full FAS occurs after alcohol exposure during the first eight weeks of embryogenesis, while exposure to alcohol later in pregnancy may affect prenatal and postnatal growth, and cause behavioural and cognitive disorders. FAS affects only one-third of those mothers who drink to such excesses. While a safe threshold of alcohol consumption has not been established, there is no evidence to suggest that levels of alcohol consumption above low-risk guidelines produce harm to the developing foetus.

A number of factors increase the likelihood of FAS – genetic factors, and factors relating to low socioeconomic status (e.g. environmental pollutants, poor nutrition, smoking, psychological stress, physical abuse). Although the prevalence of FAS is more common in minority racial groups, there is no evidence that the development of FAS is due to biological factors; drinking patterns, quantity of alcohol consumed and factors relating to low socioeconomic status are thought to contribute to the differences in expression between races. An older maternal age (30 years and over) has also been associated with the development of FAS in the child; however, this may be confounded by an increased duration of drinking rather than age per se.

DIAGNOSIS

Currently, there is no objective laboratory test for diagnosing FAS. Consequently, the diagnosis relies on both establishing the pattern of abnormalities that make up FAS, and reports (generally self-reports) of alcohol use and misuse by the mother during pregnancy and around the time of conception. Behaviour problems overlap with autism, ADHD and frontal lobe disorders.

Key features

There are three key features (*see* Box 35.1), which occur in the majority of FAS cases: growth retardation, characteristic facial features, and central nervous system anomalies or dysfunction. If an individual has abnormalities in each of the three key features, most other birth defect syndromes can be excluded, but confirmation of the diagnosis of FAS requires, in addition to symptoms, a history of maternal alcohol use during pregnancy.

BOX 35.1 Key features of foetal alcohol syndrome

1 Growth retardation associated with FAS is defined as confirmed prenatal or postnatal height or weight (or both) at or below the 10th percentile at any time.
2 Characteristic facial features of FAS are short or small palpebral fissures, thin upper lip and flattened philtrum. Other facial features are maxillary hypoplasia and epicanthal folds.
3 Central nervous system anomalies or dysfunction that occur with FAS are:
   a microcephaly (at or below the 10th percentile – but below the 3rd percentile for children with height and weight below 10th percentile)
   b clinically significant structural brain abnormalities observable through imaging techniques
   c neurological damage (such as seizures not caused by postnatal insult or fever) and soft neurological signs (e.g. coordination, nystagmus)
   d functional deficits:

either
   e global cognitive deficit – decreased IQ below expected for environment and background (the majority of individuals with FAS have an IQ around 60 to 70) or significant developmental delay (in children who are too young for an IQ assessment)

or

f   deficits in three or more of the following domains (one standard deviation below the mean on standardised tests)

g   cognitive deficits – intellectual disability and poor information processing (the individual may score in the normal range of development but below expected for environment and background)

h   executive functioning deficits (lack of inhibition, poor planning and judgement)

i   motor functioning delays or deficits (i.e. visuomotor and visuospatial coordination, delayed motor milestones, clumsiness, balance problems, poor sucking ability in infants)

j   attention and hyperactivity problems (difficulty in focusing and sustaining attention, and impulsiveness)

k   problems with social skills (social perception and social communication problems, immaturity, inappropriate sexual behaviours and interactions)

l   other problems such as sensory problems (e.g. not liking to be touched), memory deficits, language problems and unable to understand others' perspectives.

Diagnostic features can change with age. Facial features are most easily distinguishable during infancy and early preschool years, while difficulties with executive functioning and social perception skills present in children aged four to seven years.

Problems in the areas of central nervous system (CNS) function often lead to the development of maladaptive behaviour and mental health problems.

MANAGEMENT

The management of FAS involves prevention – by identifying the women who drink during pregnancy and modifying their drinking behaviour – and caring for those affected by FAS.

➤ support for families – to provide a stable home environment, parenting strategies to promote child and family functioning, and manage problem behaviours

➤ monitoring of development, and provision of early intervention for developmental and learning problems – in collaboration with services that have expertise and experience in FAS (if available)

➤ monitoring of auditory development, sensorineural and conductive hearing.

Adolescents

Even when the intellectual disability is mild or borderline families require support in parenting adolescents with FAS who require assessment and monitoring for behavioural and mental health problems such as depression, anxiety, alcohol and drug dependence, eating disorder and personality disorder. They characteristically have problems with:

➤ decision-making

➤ health and social care

➤ self-esteem

➤ concepts of time and finance.

They may present as:
➤ disrupted schooling
➤ trouble with law
➤ inappropriate sexual behaviour
➤ drug or alcohol-related problems.

Foetal alcohol spectrum disorder in adult life is associated alongside the intellectual disability and difficulties with executive function with an increased incidence of depression, bipolar disorder, anxiety, eating disorder, personality disorder and psychosis.

FURTHER READING

- Abel EL, Hannigan JH. Maternal risk factors in fetal alcohol syndrome: provocative and permissive influences. *Neurotoxicol Teratol.* 1995; **17**(4): 445–62.
- Bower C, Silva D, Henderson TR, *et al.* Ascertainment of birth defects: the effect on completeness of adding a new source of data. *J Paediatr Child Health.* 2000; **36**(6): 574–6.
- Church MW, Eldis F, Blakley BW, *et al.* Hearing, language, speech, vestibular, and dentofacial disorders in fetal alcohol syndrome. *Alcohol Clin Exp Res.* 1997; **21**(2): 227–37.
- Gerberding JL, Cordero J, Floyd RL. *Fetal Alcohol Syndrome: guidelines for referral and diagnosis.* Atlanta: National Center on Birth Defects and Developmental Disabilities, Centers for Disease Control and Prevention, National Task Force on Fetal Alcohol Syndrome; 2004.
- Jacobson JL, Jacobson SW. Drinking moderately and pregnancy: effects on child development. *Alcohol Res Health.* 1999; **23**(1): 25–30.
- Mukherjee RA, Hollins S, Turk J. Fetal alcohol spectrum disorder: an overview. *J R Soc Med.* 2006; **99**(6): 298–302.

Appendices

SUPPORT GROUPS AND ASSOCIATIONS FOR SPECIFIC SYNDROMES
Useful resources
Easyhealth
www.easyhealth.org
A tremendously useful site with information about and tailored to the needs of people with intellectual disability.

Mencap
123 Golden Lane
London
EC1Y 0RT
Tel: 020 7454 0454
Website: www.mencap.org.uk
E-mail: information@mencap.org.uk
Fax: 020 7608 3254

Support groups (UK): specific disorders
ANGELMAN SYNDROME
ASSERT (Angleman Syndrome Support Education and Research Trust)
Address (Freepost): ASSERT
PO Box 4962
Nuneaton
CV11 9FD
Tel: 0300 999 0102
Website: www.angelmanuk.org
E-mail: infro@angelmanuk.org

AUTISM SPECTRUM DISORDERS (PERVASIVE DEVELOPMENTAL DISORDERS)
Autism Care (UK)
Heath Farm
Heath Road
Scopwick

Lincolnshire
LN4 3JD
Tel: 01526 322444
Website: www.autismcareuk.com
E-mail: info@autismcareuk.com
Fax: 01526 323600

National Autistic Society
www.autism.org.uk
The website incorporates the Autism Services Directory which details resources available throughout the UK.

CEREBRAL PALSY
Scope for Cerebral Palsy and Related Disabilities
6 Market Road
London
N7 9PW
Tel: 0808 800 3333
Website: www.scope.org.uk

DOWN SYNDROME
Down's Syndrome Support Group
The Langdon Down Centre
2A Langdon Park
Teddington
Middlesex TW11 9PS
Tel: 0845 230 0372
Fax: 0845 230 0373
Website: www.downs-syndrome.org.uk
E-mail: National Office (for general enquires) info@downs-syndrome.org.uk

FRAGILE X SYNDROME
The Fragile X Society
Rood End House
6 Stortford Road
Great Dunmow
Essex CM6 1DA
Tel: 01371 875 100
Website: www.fragilex.org.uk

NEUROFIBROMATOSIS TYPE 1
The Neurofibromatosis Association
Quayside House
38 High Street
Kingston upon Thames
Surrey KT1 1HL
Tel: 020 8439 1234
Website: www.nfauk.org

E-mail: info@nfauk.org
Fax: 020 8439 1200

PRADER-WILLI SYNDROME
PWSA – Prader-Willi Syndrome Association (UK)
125a London Road
Derby
DE1 2QQ
Tel: 01332 365676
Website: www.pwsa.co.uk

RETT SYNDROME
Rett Syndrome Association
Rett UK
Langham House West
Mill Street
Luton
LU1 2NA
Tel: 01582 798910
Website: www.rettsyndrome.org.uk
E-mail: mailto:info@rettuk.org

TUBEROUS SCLEROSIS
Tuberous Sclerosis Association
PO Box 12979
Barnt Green
Birmingham
B45 5AN
Tel: 0121 445 6970
Website: www.tuberous-sclerosis.org

WILLIAMS SYNDROME
The Williams Syndrome Foundation (UK)
161 High Street
Tonbridge
Kent TN9 1BX
Tel: 01732 365152
Website: www.williams-syndrome.org.uk
E-mail: (Chief Executive: John Nelson) john.nelson@williams-syndrome.org.uk
Fax: 01732 360178

Useful websites

➤ Books Beyond Words: www.rcpsych.ac.uk/publications/booksbeyondwords.aspx
➤ British Institute of Learning Disabilities: www.bild.org.uk
➤ The 'contact a family' directory: www.cafamily.org.uk/medicalinformation/index.html (information on conditions underlying learning disabilities; medical descriptions; and details of inheritance patterns and prenatal diagnosis).

- Down Syndrome Medical Interest Group: www.dsmig.org.uk
- Foundation for People with Learning Disabilities: www.learningdisabilities. org.uk/
- Learning Disability Coalition: Learning about Intellectual Disabilities and Health, a web-based learning resource: www.learningdisabilitycoalition.org.uk
- Newcastle University: www.ncl.ac.uk/nnp/teaching/resources/learning.pdf
- National Association for Down Syndrome: www.nads.org
- SENSE: www.sense.org.uk (SENSE is the leading national charity that supports and campaigns for children and adults who are deafblind).
- Skill: www.skill.org.uk (promoting equality in education, training and employment for disabled people).
- Understanding Intellectual Disability and Health: www.intellectualdisability. info

Glossary

The glossary is compiled primarily to assist readers who do not have an extensive medical knowledge. For more detailed descriptions of terms, consult a medical dictionary or other specialist information.

abdominal obstruction   blockage of the bowel (gut), which causes pain

aetiology   causes of the disease, disorder or disability

akathisia   long-term or persistent condition of motor restlessness which may present as being unable to sit or lie quietly, or sleep

amenorrhoea   absence of menstruation

amniocentesis   obtaining amniotic fluid for genetic testing from around the foetus (baby) in the uterus

anticholinergic effects   desired or undesired effects of medication which may include a dry mouth, fast heart rate, blurred vision, constipation, sweating and hot flushes

antiepileptics   medication for management of fits, seizures or convulsions

anxiolytics   medication used to induce calm by treating/reducing anxiety

aortic stenosis   narrowing or obstruction of the great artery that leads from the left ventricle of the heart

Apgar scores   numerical expression of the condition of a newborn baby, calculated soon after birth, which considers heart rate, breathing effort, muscle tone, reflexes and colour

applied behaviour analysis (ABA)   investigation of environmental factors that affect behaviour; analysis of events that occur for, or as a consequence of, a specific behaviour

arterial stenosis   narrowing or blocking of arteries

asphyxia   suffocation, often through blockage of the airways

aspiration pneumonia   infection of the lungs caused by aspiration of food or other foreign material

aspiration   breathing in or inhaling; also the removal of fluid or gases from the body using suction

asymmetrical septal hypertrophy   abnormally enlarged heart muscle situated between the left and right side of the heart

ataxia   problem with muscular coordination often causing clumsiness or difficulty walking

athetosis involuntary continuous writhing movements, especially severe in the hands

atlantoaxial instability laxity of the ligaments attached to the vertebral bones in the upper neck

atrial septal defect defect in the dividing wall between the upper chambers of the heart

Bayley Scale of Infant Development a scale used to assess development in children

behavioural intervention plan planned or systematic response to a person's behaviour, with the aim of changing the behaviour

bioavailability the degree to which a drug or other substance becomes available to the target tissue after administration

bipolar affective disorder severe disorder of mood, often involving recurrent depression and at least one episode of abnormally elevated mood

birth asphyxia lack of oxygen that, unless remedied, can lead to suffocation and death

café au lait spots light-brown coloured skin markings

cardiovascular relating to the heart and blood vessels

catamenial epilepsy epilepsy associated with the menstrual cycle

cerebrovascular relating to the blood vessels of the brain

challenging behaviour behaviour which recurs and is substantially disruptive to the individual and other people; it may limit the individual's capacity to learn, and the safety of the individual, others and the community

chorionic villus sampling test in early pregnancy where a sample of the placenta is removed for analysis

coarctation a narrowing of vessels

cognitive disintegration decline in intellectual functioning where aspects of thinking and perception begin to break down or fail

comorbidity diseases found together with a syndrome or disorder, not necessarily biologically related to the syndrome or disorder

computerised tomography (CT) a scan that produces a two-dimensional image of the body using multiple X-rays and a computer

congenital heart disease heart disease existing from birth

consent agreement, compliance and permission following understanding and insight

contractures condition of fixed high resistance to stretching of muscles, leading to deformities that do not allow extension of joints

cryptoorchidism undescended testes or testes not in the scrotum

cubitus vulgus deformity of the elbow with sideways deviation of the forearm (judged when the palm of the hand faces forward)

cytogenetic testing genetic testing which examines chromosomes that are associated with heredity; can determine chances of families carrying particular conditions/ diseases in their genes

cytomegalovirus (CMV) virus which can cause abnormalities in the foetus

Denver II test a test used to assess children with developmental delay

deoxyribonucleic acid (DNA) test scientific testing of the substance found in all living cells which is the carrier of all genetic information, used to identify disabling conditions and determine carriage of the condition in future pregnancies and generations

depot formulation of medication for injection into a muscle, designed to release slowly (usually over a period of months)

developmental disability delayed milestones occurring during childhood, usually before school age; may be influenced by an intellectual or physical impairment, environmental factors or a combination

developmental syndromes   particular conditions with identifiable characteristics or needs, which are usually first diagnosed in childhood

diagnostic overshadowing   a situation where one condition masks or hides another condition or symptom

differential diagnosis   the determination of which one of two or more diseases or conditions a patient is suffering from, by systematically comparing and contrasting their clinical findings

diplegia   bilateral paralysis; paralysis affecting both sides of the body

dislocation   displacement of any part, usually the end of bone being pushed out of a joint

drug excretion   medication being eliminated/removed from the body, usually through urine or faeces

drug metabolism   the chemical processes involved in a drug being altered within the body

ductus arteriosus   persistent problem after birth where blood flows from the aorta to the pulmonary artery and there is recirculation of arterial blood through the lungs

dysarthria   problem with speech articulation due to disturbances in muscular control relating to central nervous system (CNS) damage

dysmorphic features   features that appear different from the ordinary

dysplasia   abnormal development

dyspraxia   coordination difficulties

dystonia   disordered muscle tone

dystonic reactions   faulty or malplaced muscle reactions

echolalia   repetition of words or phrases

ecology of the family   consideration of the many factors affecting the family, including psychosocial factors

elastin disorder   problem with elastin (the essential part of connective tissue)

electroencephalogram (EEG)   non-invasive recording of electrical energy of the brain; often used to assess epilepsy

endometrial ablation   surgical removal of the lining of the uterus

epicanthal fold   a vertical fold of skin between the nose and the eye

epiloia   tuberous sclerosis

equinus deformity   talipes equinus (or clubfoot); deformity of the foot present at birth, where the foot is twisted out of shape (plantar flexed), causing the person to walk on the toes without the heel touching the ground

expressive communication   usually speech, but can involve facial and body expressions

extrapyramidal effects   often medication-related adverse effects which affect voluntary control over skilled movements, particularly tongue (speech), hands and feet

facilitated communication   communication that may be assisted by devices such as a communication board, computer or another person providing physical assistance

fibroma   a benign tumour made up of fibrous or connective tissue

gait apraxia   problems with the manner or style of walking, despite there being no paralysis

gastro-oesophageal dysfunction   problems associated with the stomach and the oesophagus

gastrostomy   a surgical creation of an artificial opening between the abdominal wall (on the outside) and the stomach; often made to allow direct feeding to enhance the nutritional status of the person

genes   contain information that codes an individual's genetic make-up; genetic material is passed on from generation to generation

geneticist   specialist medical practitioner who works with genes and the study of problems associated with human heredity

genitourinary problem   problems associated with the genital and urinary organs

gingival hypertrophy   enlargement and overgrowth of the gums

glioma   a type of brain tumour

global delay   developmental delay affecting all areas of growth and development in the child under school age

Griffiths Mental Development Scales   scales used to measure the rate of development of infants and children to eight years

guardianship   legal process, by which a designated person is authorised to make substituted decisions on behalf of another person; authenticates the role of a proxy decision-maker

gynaecomastia   excessive development of the male breasts

habilitation   the process of enabling people with disability to develop skills to allow them to participate fully in the community

Helicobacter pylori   a bacteria associated with peptic ulcer disease; it occurs more commonly in people who reside in institutions and those with poor oral hygiene

hemiparesis   muscular weakness affecting only one side of the body

hemiplegia   paralysis of one side of the body

homeostasis   a tendency to stabilise normal body states, brought about by complex chemical controls

hyperacusis   an exceptionally good sense of hearing; painful sensitivity to sound

hyperandrogenism   a state caused by excessive levels of androgen hormones in the body

hyperextensible joints   joints that can be extended further than is usual

hypergraphia   writing a lot

hyperphagia   overeating; ingestion of excessive amounts of food

hyperprolactinaemia   high levels of the hormone prolactin in the blood; may be due to medication (particularly antipsychotics), breastfeeding or a tumour

hypertelorism   abnormally spaced distance between two body parts or organs (e.g. the eyes)

hypocalcaemia   a shortage of calcium in the blood

hypogonadism   abnormally decreased function of the gonads (i.e. testes or ovaries) resulting in significantly delayed growth and sexual development

hypomania   mania of a moderate type

hypopigmented skin   abnormally diminished skin pigmentation (colouring of the skin)

hypotonia   diminished tone of the muscles (e.g. a limb that becomes floppy)

hypoxia   low oxygen content in the tissues

immunodeficiency   deficiency in the immune response (reaction of the body to fight infection)

inguinal hernia   part of a body organ which protrudes and becomes visible in the groin area, causing pain and potentially obstruction of the bowel

intellectual disability   refers to limitations in intellectual functioning (e.g. difficulty in learning and performing certain daily life skills); usually evident before the age of 18 years

ischaemic encephalopathy   any degenerative disease of the brain caused by constriction or obstruction of blood supply

karyotype   chromosomal make-up of a person

kyphosis   hunchback; abnormally increased curvature of the spine when viewed from the side

magnetic resonance imaging (MRI)   non-invasive imaging of the body using magnetic energy to produce multidimensional pictures

malar hypoplasia   incomplete development of the cheek or cheekbone (does not reach adult size)

malignant   tending to become worse and result in death

malocclusion   improper positioning of the teeth and jaws; commonly called 'bad bite'

mandibular prognathism   marked protrusion or jutting out of the lower jaw

mania   an abnormal mental state marked by an extended emotional state which may include elation, increased activity and talkativeness

maternal serum screening   blood tests in pregnancy to check for problems with the baby or mother

maxillary hypoplasia   underdevelopment of the upper jaw

menorrhoea   menstruation; period

microcephaly   abnormally small size of the head; usually accompanied by intellectual disability

micrognathia   unusually small size of the jaw

monotherapy   treatment of a condition or disease using only one medication

mood-congruent delusions   false beliefs that cannot be corrected by fact or objective reasoning, but are consistent with the person's mood

morbidity   conditions associated with a disease

mortality   death, often expressed as mortality rates or death rates

mutation   a change in form, quality or other characteristic; often used to refer to changes in gene structure which may result in a specific disease or a cluster of specific physical characteristics known as a syndrome (e.g. Down syndrome)

myopia   near-sightedness (also called short-sightedness); requiring glasses to see long distances clearly

nasogastric feeding   when specially prepared food is introduced directly to the stomach through a tube that is inserted through the nose and down the canal that leads to the stomach

neonatal   associated with a baby in the first four weeks after birth

neuroimaging   sensitive non-invasive technology to view or map the brain (e.g. MRI and CT scans)

neurological adverse effects   adverse effects of medication that have an effect on the central nervous system and/or cognitive function (e.g. dizziness, sedation)

non-pharmacological management   treatments and management other than drugs

nystagmus   a fast, involuntary movement of the eye

oesophagitis   inflammation of the oesophagus

oesophagus   the tube that connects the mouth to the stomach

orthoses   physical aids and assistive devices (such as splints, braces) which are used to support, align and improve the function of moveable body parts; used as corrective and preventive devices

osteopenia   reduced bone mass

osteoporosis   demineralisation of bone resulting in loss of bone density (mass); often found in older people and people with disability; can lead to physical bone fractures

otoscopy   ear examination using a special instrument

paediatrics   the specialist branch of medicine that studies and treats childhood diseases and illnesses

palmar   relating to the palm of the hand

palpebral fissures   the corners of the eyes and associated eyelids

parkinsonian effects   a specific group of central nervous system adverse drug effects including decreased mobility, tremor, stiff and inflexible muscles

pectus carinatum   chicken or pigeon chest; prominence (sticking out) of the breast area (sternum)

pectus excavatum   funnel chest; hollowed-out, depressed breast area (sternum)

periorbital fullness   swelling around the eye socket

pes planus   deformity of the foot so that the arch of the foot is lowered, resulting in a flatfoot appearance

phenotype   the entire physical, biochemical and physiological make-up of a person, as determined both genetically and environmentally

philtrum   the vertical groove in the middle of the upper lip

plexiform   resembling a network

polycystic ovaries   ovaries (female egg-producing organs) that contain many cysts

polypharmacy   use of multiple medications at the same time

postural hypotension   low blood pressure made worse by moving to a standing position

precocious puberty   sexual maturity in a child that occurs earlier than the usual age

premutation   having a defect in a gene, but does not cause symptoms

presbycusis   hearing loss in both ears that occurs with age

prn medication   (prn = *pro re nata*: 'as the thing is needed') medication prescribed by a medical practitioner to be given on an as needed basis; often given in response to particular events taking place (e.g. sedation for someone who is agitated)

pseudarthrosis   bending and fracture of a long bone which does not heal, and thus creates a 'false joint'

pseudopsychotic presentations   actions or reactions that mimic or replicate psychosis

psychometric testing   measurement of intellectual processes including comprehension, memory, understanding and analytical ability, usually carried out by a psychologist; a number of standard (regulated) tests are used

psychosis   a term used to describe a major mental health condition where the person loses contact with reality, often with delusions, hallucinations or illusions

psychotherapy   a talking-based therapy using intellectual reasoning rather than a pharmacological or medicine-driven approach; therapy to help the individual understand their problems and address often deep-seated or past events that affect current behaviour and attitudes

ptosis   drooping of the upper eyelid in response to nerve paralysis

pulmonary valvular stenosis   blockage or restriction in the outlet valve of the right side of the heart

quadriplegia   tetraplegia; paralysis of all four limbs

receptive communication   ability to understand and comprehend information

rhabdomyomata of the heart   benign tumours of the heart that have muscular elements

scoliosis   sideways curvature of the spine

seizure   a fit or convulsion

sleep apnoea   when breathing stops during sleep; can lead to asphyxia

spermatogenesis   production of sperm

static brain insult   single episode of injury to the brain

status epilepticus   series of rapid and repeated epileptic fits or convulsions during which the person is unconscious

stellate irides   where each iris (the coloured part of the eye surrounding the pupil) is shaped like a star

stenosis   an abnormal narrowing

stereotypic movement disorder   a disorder characterised by continuous and repetitive movements that are not purposeful; the movements may be restrictive and inflexible in intensity or focus (e.g. hand-flapping, rocking)

strabismus   squint; when both eyes appear to look in different directions

subluxation   an incomplete or partial dislocation

talipes equinovarus   typical clubfoot; a deformity of the foot where the heel is turned inwards from the midline of the leg and the foot is plantar-flexed (toes pointing downwards)

tardive dyskinesia   impairment of the power of voluntary movement often associated with long-term administration of antipsychotics

thrombophlebitis   inflammation associated with the vein where a blood clot forms or lodges

topographically invariant motor skills   repetitive, potentially injurious behaviour such as head-banging, flicking of fingers or hands, that has no logical purpose

toxic levels   when the amount of a particular medication is too much

toxoplasmosis   a disease which can be transmitted to the baby in the womb; it can lead to major problems with the central nervous system including blindness, brain defects and death

vasculopathy   a disorder of the blood vessels

vasomotor instability   over-reactivity of the blood vessels

visuomotor   relating to the coordination of sight and movement

visuospatial   relating to the coordination of sight and space

WISC-IV test   Wechsler Intelligence Scale for Children (edition 4) – a standardised psychological test designed to assess intellectual functioning in children aged five to 15

xerostomia   dry mouth

Index